Pesticide residues in food - 1985

FAO
PLANT
PRODUCTION
AND PROTECTION
PAPER

68

Report of the Joint Meeting of the
FAO Panel of Experts on Pesticide Residues
in Food and the Environment
and a WHO Expert Group on Pesticide Residues
Geneva, 23 September - 2 October 1985

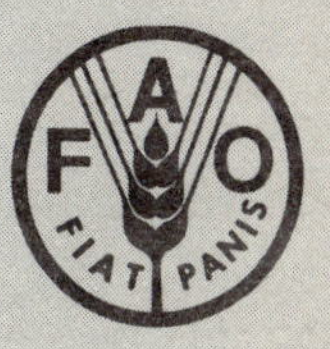

FOOD
AND
AGRICULTURE
ORGANIZATION
OF THE
UNITED NATIONS
Rome, 1986

Monographs containing summaries of residue data and toxicological data considered at the 1985 JMPR, together with recommendations, are available upon request from FAO under the title:

Pesticide residues in food - 1985
Evaluations 1985
FAO Plant Production and Protection Paper

The designations employed and the presentation of material in this publication do not imply the expression of any opinion whatsoever on the part of the Food and Agriculture Organization of the United Nations concerning the legal status of any country, territory, city or area or of its authorities, or concerning the delimitation of its frontiers or boundaries.

This report contains the collective views of two international groups of experts and does not necessarily represent the decisions or the stated policy of the Food and Agriculture Organization of the United Nations or of the World Health Organization.

INTERNATIONAL PROGRAMME ON CHEMICAL SAFETY

The preparatory work for the toxicological evaluations of pesticide residues carried out by the WHO Expert Group on Pesticide Residues for consideration by the FAO/WHO Joint Meeting on Pesticide Residues in Food and the Environment is actively supported by the International Programme on Chemical Safety (IPCS).
The International Programme on Chemical Safety (IPCS) is a joint venture of the United Nations Environment Programme, the International Labour Organisation, and the World Health Organization. One of the main objectives of the IPCS is to carry out and disseminate evaluations of the effects of chemicals on human health and the quality of the environment.

M-84
ISBN 92-5-102365-4

TABLE OF CONTENTS

([1]) R = Residues; T = Toxicology

---

* Compounds re-evaluated by the present meeting

1985 JOINT MEETING OF THE FAO PANEL OF EXPERTS ON PESTICIDE RESIDUES
IN FOOD AND THE ENVIRONMENT AND THE WHO EXPERT GROUP ON
PESTICIDE RESIDUES

Geneva, 23 September - 2 October 1985

FAO Panel of Experts on Pesticide Residues in Food and the Environment

Dr D.C. Abbott, Ashtead, United Kingdom (Rapporteur).

Mr J.A.R. Bates, Head, Pesticide Registration Department, Ministry of
Agriculture, Fisheries and Food, Harpenden, United Kingdom (Vice-Chairman).

Professor Dr A.F.H. Besemer, formerly Chair of Phytopharmacy, Agricultural
University, Wageningen, The Netherlands.

Dr E. Celma-Calamita, Ministerio de Agricultura, Pesca y Alimentacion,
Madrid, Spain.

Mr N.F. Ives, Environmental Protection Agency, Office of Pesticide Programs,
Washington, D.C., USA.

Mr K. Voldum-Clausen, Division of Pesticides and Contaminants, National Food
Agency, Soborg, Denmark.

Observers invited by FAO

Dr W. Bosse, GTZ Pesticide Residue Laboratory, Darmstadt, Federal Republic of
Germany.

Mr A.J. Pieters, Ministry of Welfare, Health and Cultural Affairs,
Leidschendam, The Netherlands.

WHO Expert Group on Pesticide Residues

Dr V. Benes, Chief, Department of Toxicology, Institute of Hygiene and
Epidemiology, Prague, Czechoslovakia.

Mr D.J. Clegg, Head, Pesticide Section, Toxicological Evaluation Division,
Food Directorate, Health Protection Branch, Ottawa, Canada (Chairman).

Dr A.H. El-Sebae, Chairman, Pesticides Division, Faculty of Agriculture,
Alexandria University, Alexandria, Egypt.

Professor M. Lotti, Professor of Industrial Toxicology, Istituto di
Medicina del Lavoro, Padua, Italy.

Dr O.E. Paynter, Chief Scientist, Hazard Evaluation Division, US Environmental
Protection Agency, Washington, D.C., USA.

Professor T.J. Pekkanen, Head, Department of Food and Environmental Hygiene,
College of Veterinary Medicine, Helsinki, Finland.

Professor R. Plestina, Head, Department of Toxicology, Institute for Medical
Research and Occupational Health, Zagreb, Yugoslavia.

Professor F.G. Reyes, Faculdade de Engenharia de Alimentos, Universidade
     Estadual de Campinas, Campinas SP, Brazil (Rapporteur).

Secretariat

Dr A.L. Black, Medical Services Adviser, Commonwealth Department of Health
    Woden, Australia   (WHO Temporary Adviser),

Dr E. Budd, Supervisory Toxicologist, Hazard Evaluation Division,
     US Environmental Protection Agency, Washington, D.C., USA (WHO Temporary
     Adviser).

Dr J.R.P. Cabral, Unit of Mechanisms of Carcinogenesis, International Agency
     for Research on Cancer, Lyon, France.   (WHO Temporary Adviser).

Dr A. Di Muccio, Research Officer, Laboratorio Tossicologia Applicata,
     Istituto Superiore di Sanità, Rome, Italy (WHO Temporary Adviser).

Dr M. Gilbert, Scientific Affairs Officer, IRPTC/UNEP, Geneva, Switzerland
    (WHO Temporary Adviser).

Dr H. Galal Gorchev, Food Safety, Division of Environmental Health,
    WHO, Geneva, Switzerland.

Dr J.L. Herrman, Center for Food Safety and Applied Nutrition, Food and
    Drug Administration, Washington, D.C., USA (WHO Consultant).

Mr G. van den Hurk, Technical Officer, International Programme on Chemical
    Safety, Division of Environmental Health, WHO, Geneva, Switzerland.

Dr R.B. Jaeger, Section Head, Toxicology Branch, Hazard Evaluation Division,
    US Environmental Protection Agency, Washington, D.C., USA (WHO Temporary
    Adviser).

Dr F.K. Kaeferstein, Manager, Food Safety, Division of Environmental Health,
    WHO, Geneva, Switzerland.

Dr F.-W. Kopisch-Obuch, Pesticide Residues Specialist, Plant Protection
    Service,
    Food and Agriculture Organization, Rome, Italy (Joint Secretary).

Dr L.G. Ladomery, Food Standards Officer, Joint FAO/WHO Food Standards
    Programme, Food and Agriculture Organization, Rome, Italy.

Mr A.F. Machin, London, United Kingdom (FAO Consultant).

Dr M. Mercier, Manager, International Programme on Chemical Safety, Division
    of Environmental Health, WHO, Geneva, Switzerland.

Dr A. Pelfrène, Pesticides Development and Safe Use, Division of Vector
    Biology and Control, WHO, Geneva, Switzerland.

Mr J.R. Plimmer, Head, Agrochemicals and Residues Section, Joint FAO/IAEA
    Division, IAEA, Vienna, Austria.

Professor A. Rico, Director, Laboratoire de Toxicologie Biochimique et
Metabolique, (I.N.R.A.), Ecole National Vétérinaire, <u>Toulouse</u>,
France   (WHO Temporary Adviser).

Professor V. Silano, Director, Department of Comparative Toxicology and
Ecotoxicology, Istituto Superiore di Sanità, <u>Rome</u>, Italy (WHO
Temporary Adviser).

Dr A. Takanaka, Head, Division of Pharmacology, Biological Safety Research
Center, National Institute of Hygienic Sciences, <u>Tokyo</u>, Japan (WHO
Temporary Adviser).

Professor K. Topsy, Member Pesticide Control Board, Ministry of Health,
<u>Beau Bassin</u>, Mauritius   (WHO Temporary Adviser).

Dr G. Vettorazzi, Senior Toxicologist, International Programme on Chemical
Safety, Division of Environmental Health, WHO, <u>Geneva</u>, Switzerland
(Joint Secretary).

Dr D. Wu-Lau, Scientific Adviser, Toxicological Evaluation Division, Food
Directorate, Health Protection Branch, <u>Ottawa</u>, Canada (WHO Temporary
Adviser).

Mr J.R. Wessel, Director, Contaminants Policy Staff, Office of Regulatory
Affairs, Food and Drug Administration, Rockville, <u>Maryland</u>, USA.

ABBREVIATIONS AND ACRONYMS
(Does not include chemical abbreviations)

ADI: Acceptable Daily Intake

ai: active ingredient

bw: body weight

CAC: Codex Alimentarius Commission

CCPR: Codex Committee on Pesticide Residues

EDI: Estimated Daily Intake

ERL: Extraneous Residue Limit

FAO: Food and Agriculture Organization of the United Nations

g: gram

GAP: Good Agricultural Practice

GI: Gastro-Intestinal

GL: Guideline Level

GLC: Gas-Liquid Chromatography

ha: hectare

IAEA: International Atomic Energy Agency - FAO

IARC: International Agency for Research on Cancer

IPCS: International Programme on Chemical Safety

IRPTC: International Register of Potentially Toxic Chemicals

JMPR: Joint Meeting on Pesticide Residues (Joint Meeting of the FAO Panel of Experts on Pesticide Residues in Food and the Environment and the WHO Expert Group on Pesticide Residues)

kg: kilogram

l: litre

LD_{50}:   Lethal Dose, median

mg: Milligram

MRL**:   Residue levels at or about the limit of determination

MRL: Maximum Residue Limit

NCI: National Cancer Institute (United States)

NOEL: No Observed Effect Level

PHI: Pre-Harvest Interval

ppm: parts per million

SCE: Sister Chromatid Exchange

TADI: Temporary Acceptable Daily Intake

TDI: Theoretical Daily Intake

TMRL: Temporary Maximum Residue Limit (Note: This term replaces "tolerance")

UNEP: United Nations Environment Programme

WHO: World Health Organization of the United Nations

PESTICIDE RESIDUES IN FOOD

Report of the 1985 Joint FAO/WHO Meeting of Experts

A joint meeting of the FAO Panel of Experts on Pesticide Residues in Food and the Environment and the WHO Expert Group on Pesticide Residues (JMPR) was held in Geneva, Switzerland, from 23 September to 2 October 1985. The meeting was opened by Dr J. Hamon, Assistant Director-General of WHO, on behalf of the Directors-General of FAO and WHO. The FAO Panel had already met in preparatory sessions on 19 and 20 September.

After thanking all participants for having accepted the invitation to contribute to the work of the 1985 joint meeting, Dr Hamon indicated the importance of pesticides in controlling pests and diseases and the essential role of the joint meeting in assessing and minimizing the health hazards posed by pesticide residues in food.

Dr Hamon stated that the importance of this work was recently recognized by the inter-country meeting ("The Evaluation of Pesticide Residues in Food - The Need to Accelerate International Action") held in Canada, in April 1985, that produced a number of valuable recommendations to strengthen the long and distinguished record of the JMPR. Several actions had already been taken by the International Programme on Chemical Safety (IPCS) to implement these recommendations. They included the organization of a meeting to update the principles and methodology to assess pesticide residues in food, the elaboration of guidelines for evaluating biological agents used as pesticides, the development of criteria for cyclic re-evaluation of pesticides, the establishment of a two-year cycle for evaluation of compounds by the JMPR, and several steps to improve the dissemination and visibility of the deliberations of the JMPR.

Dr Hamon also informed the meeting of the death of Professor Emilio Astolfi of Argentina in July 1985 and expressed his deep regret. He called for a minute of silence in his memory. Professor Astolfi, a toxicologist of international reputation, made very valuable contributions to the work of the joint meetings for a number of years.

1. INTRODUCTION

The meeting was held in pursuance of recommendations made by previous meetings and accepted by the governing bodies of FAO and WHO that studies should be undertaken jointly by experts to evaluate possible hazards to man arising from the occurrence of residues of pesticides in foods. The reports of previous joint meetings (see references, Section 7) contain information on acceptable daily intakes for man (ADIs), maximum residue limits (MRLs) and general principles of evaluation for the various pesticides considered. The supporting documents contain detailed monographs on these pesticides and include comments on analytical methods. The present meeting was convened to consider a further number of pesticides together with items of a general or a specific nature. These included items for clarification of recommendations made at previous meetings or for reconsideration of previous evaluations in the light of findings of subsequent research or other developments.

During the meeting the FAO Panel of Experts was responsible for reviewing pesticide use patterns (good agricultural practice), data on the chemistry and composition of pesticides and methods of analysis of pesticide residues and for estimating the maximum residue levels that might occur following the use of the pesticide according to good agricultural practice. The WHO Expert Group was responsible for reviewing toxicological and related data and for estimating, where possible, ADIs for man for the pesticides. The recommendations of the joint meeting, including further research and information, are proposed for use by Member Governments of the respective agencies and other interested parties.

2. GENERAL CONSIDERATIONS

2.1 MODIFICATIONS TO THE AGENDA

The meeting deferred consideration of chinomethionat, clofentezine and phenothrin to a future meeting because no data were submitted.

Several questions raised at the 17th Session of the CCPR were considered. These are listed in Section 2.8

2.2 GENERAL PRINCIPLES FOR ESTIMATING ADIs

The meeting took account of the principles elaborated in the reports of previous meetings (see Section 7 of this Report) concerning the estimation of ADIs and the formulation of other decisions based on toxicological considerations. In particular, it endorsed the opinions expressed by the 1978, 1982 and 1983 JMPRs and reaffirmed its general adherence to those principles.

It also took account of a number of reports of other committees, in particular the principles and guidelines contained in the Seventeenth Report of the Joint FAO/WHO Expert Committee on Food Additives,[1] the report of the WHO Scientific Group on Procedures for Investigating Intentional Food Additives[2] and the report of the WHO Scientific Group on Assessment of the Carcinogenicity and Mutagenicity of Chemicals[3].

The estimation of ADIs requires a review of all pertinent available toxicological data. The extent and sufficiency of these data are major factors in the estimation of an ADI or temporary ADI, or the decision to withdraw an ADI, full or temporary.

The estimation of the hazard of pesticide residues follows an established pattern: collection of adequate and appropriate data, validation of the reliability of the data, its toxicological review and finally evaluation of that review to permit estimation of a level of dietary exposure which is unlikely to result in harm to man. It should be appreciated that the bulk of the toxicological data on pesticides traditionally considered by the JMPR are, and are likely to remain, unpublished. These data ordinarily include proprietary data as well as information submitted by governments and other interested parties. Also, whenever available, relevant published reports from the open literature are considered.

---

[1] WHO, Technical Report Series, No. 539; FAO Nutrition Meetings Report Series, No. 53, 1974.
[2] WHO, Technical Report Series, No 348, 1967.
[3] WHO, Technical Report Series, No. 546, 1974.

2.3 ISSUES RELATED TO TESTING FOR CARCINOGENICITY

The joint meeting reiterated the view expressed at previous meetings (e.g. JMPR 1983 and 1984) that the enhancement of common spontaneously-occurring liver tumours by a chemical in certain strains of mice, but not in other species, may carry less weight than other findings. In view of current knowledge of biochemical and/or genetic peculiarities underlying the induction of liver tumours in mice, the meeting deemed it unwise to consider a substance as a carcinogen solely on this type of evidence. Moreover, when a chemical increases the incidence of liver tumours in mice, carcinogenicity studies in species other than the mouse should be indicated.

The meeting noted that some of the available oncogenicity studies in mice did not include haematology. Such studies can be acceptable as carcino-genicity investigations provided they had been properly designed and executed with comprehensive histopathological examinations. However, the meeting recommended that haematology determinations in future oncogenicity studies in mice should be performed at least at termination.

2.4 ONCOGENIC METABOLITES

In evaluating diflubenzuron and thiodicarb, the joint meeting discussed whether pesticides which do not show, upon adequate testing, any carcinogenic potential, but are known to yield metabolite(s) found to be potentially oncogenic in their own right, would require any special studies to assess more in depth the health significance of the metabolite(s). While stressing that every pesticide should be evaluated on an individual basis, the meeting concluded that no special reasons for concern need to be attached to these metabolite(s) provided sufficient data are available to rule out the possibility of their occurrence in significant concentrations in food.

2.5 AVAILABILITY OF DOCUMENTS RESULTING FROM JOINT MEETINGS

Concern has been expressed at the availability of the reports of the JMPR and the associated evaluations. Currently, the documents are distributed by FAO to Ministries of Agriculture, national Codex contact points and other bodies as they become available. However, this does not always ensure their availability to Ministries of Health and the Environment or to interested institutions and individuals. Therefore the meeting recommended that the current mode of distribution of JMPR reports and evaluations be examined, and where appropriate revised, in order to ensure their receipt by all the relevant ministries and their availability to interested institutions and individuals. This revision should also be undertaken with the aim of increasing the visibility of the work of the JMPR.

2.6 QUALITY OF TOXICOLOGICAL DATA

Problems with the quality of toxicological data have been considered in the past by the 1980, 1981 and 1984 JMPRs. They continue.

In particular, the WHO Expert Group on Pesticide Residues considered at length the toxicological basis and data requirements for estimation of an ADI and a temporary ADI, and to provide general guidance on relevant toxicological methodology.

The meeting recommended that these issues be considered by an international meeting and subsequently placed on the agenda of the next joint meeting.

2.7. REVISED CODEX CLASSIFICATION OF FOODS AND ANIMAL FEEDSTUFFS

The CCPR at its 17th Session considered the revised classification (CAC/PR 4 - 1984, Preliminary Issue) and requested the JMPR to consider it also.

A second, slightly amended, edition of the revision (CAC/PR 4 - 1985, Preliminary Issue) was available to the present meeting, and was used as far as possible as the basis for commodity descriptions in estimating maximum residue levels. The new Commodity Classification Numbers are linked to the commodities listed in Annex I to this report.

2.8 REPORT OF THE 17TH SESSION OF THE CODEX COMMITTEE ON PESTICIDE RESIDUES (ALINORM 85/24 B)

The meeting noted the report of the 17th Session of the CCPR, in particular those paragraphs in which the CCPR had drawn certain items to the attention of the JMPR. Several of these were considered at the meeting and are dealt with in Sections 2, 3 and 4. Items of a general nature were:

MRLs, ADIs and assessment of consumer risk (para 220); see 2.9.
Revised Codex Classification of foods and animal feedstuffs (para 188); see 2.7.

MRLs for fumigants in the absence of an ADI (para 164 and ALINORM 85/24A, paras 236-247). The meeting deferred discussion on this item until 1986, owing to lack of time.

MRLs for ethylenethiourea (ETU) (para 173 and ALINORM 85/24A, paras 261-263). The meeting also deferred discussion on this item until 1986 owing to lack of time.

Questions on the following individual compounds were also considered:

fenvalerate (para 28); see 4.30
diphenylamine (para 33). The meeting noted that the question was discussed in the 1984 evaluations and did not consider it further.
chinomethionat (para 92). The meeting did not consider this item because the data requested by the 1981 meeting have not been submitted.
dialifos (para 102); see 4.19
dithiocarbamate fungicides (para 113); see 4.25
aldicarb (para 123); see 4.1
cypermethrin (para 128); see 4.16
permethrin (paras 134, 136); see 4.42
isofenphos (para 151); see 4.34
triadimefon (para 153); see 4.54
deltamethrin (paras 156, 157); see 4.18
metalaxyl (paras 160, 161); see 4.36
bromomethane (para 164); see 4.5

2.9 MRLs, ADIs AND ASSESSMENT OF CONSUMER RISK

The meeting was of the opinion that there was a general lack of understanding of the procedures used by the JMPR in estimating MRLs and ADIs, the objectives of these estimates, and their application in the assessment of consumer risk. It recommended that efforts be made to increase the general awareness of the work of the JMPR and to improve understanding of the ways in which MRLs and ADIs can be used in a scientifically acceptable manner.

A discussion paper "Codex Limits for Pesticide Residues in Food and Consumer Safety" prepared by the CCPR Working Group on Regulatory Principles, a revised version to be presented to the 18th Session of the CCPR, was examined by the meeting. There was general agreement with the view expressed in the paper that it was important to proceed quickly to develop guidance for those seeking assurance that adherence to maximum residue limits in individual commodities contributes to ensuring the safety of food to consumers.

The meeting supported the proposal in the discussion paper which recommended that a special joint FAO/WHO meeting should be convened to develop the required guidance. The meeting further recommended that the procedures outlined in the discussion paper, using the concepts of theoretical daily intake (TDI) and estimated daily intake (EDI) to estimate potential dietary exposure to pesticide residues should be explored together with other relevant procedures which could contribute to a better appreciation of the issues involved. The meeting also recommended that it is essential that this matter be considered in full detail at the next JMPR.

2.10 GUIDELINES ON SUPERVISED TRIALS TO PROVIDE DATA ON THE NATURE AND AMOUNT OF PESTICIDE RESIDUES IN FOODS OF ANIMAL ORIGIN

The meeting was informed of the above guidelines which had been developed by the CCPR Ad Hoc Working Group on Development of Residues Data and Sampling. These guidelines were welcomed as a valuable contribution which should improve the quality of the residue data on foods of animal origin. The Meeting noted that consideration of the principles involved in interpreting animal transfer studies in conjunction with realistic estimates of the intake of pesticide residues by animals was urgently needed and proposed to study the problem at the next meeting (see paragraph 4.28 of 1984 JMPR report).

The meeting was informed that publication of the guidelines would be arranged by FAO, Rome.

3. SPECIFIC PROBLEMS

3.1 CYHEXATIN/AZOCYCLOTIN

Since the JMPR first reviewed azocylotin (the 1,2,4-triazole derivative of cyhexatin) in 1979 it has been clear that residues at harvest resulting from the use of azocylotin and cyhexatin cannot be distinguished analytically. The only way a use of azocylotin could be confirmed by the analysis of residues would be on a sample taken soon after the application of the compound.

The current preferred analytical method converts both azocylotin and cyhexatin to tricyclohexylmethyltin and in 1982 the JMPR proposed new definitions for the residues from both compounds as follows:

<u>Cyhexatin</u> – the sum of cyhexatin and dicyclohexyltin oxide expressed as cyhexatin.

<u>Azocylotin</u> – the sum of azocylotin, cyhexatin and dicyclohexyltin oxide expressed as cyhexatin.

After re-examining the available information and taking into account the discussions on the subject at the 15th and 16th Sessions of the CCPR (1983 and 1984), the meeting recognized the possibility of administrative difficulties arising from the different registered uses of the two compounds in some countries. However, bearing in mind the current good agricultural practices in the use of the compounds, in particular the intervals between application and harvest, and the analytical problems facing regulatory authorities, the meeting concluded that the best way of presenting the MRLs for these two compounds would be in a single list. The meeting considered that it is essential to indicate clearly which parent compound had been applied in developing the residue data on which each MRL was based. For apples, beans and strawberries, the MRLs take into account the residues data derived from uses of both cyhexatin and azocyclotin.

Attention is drawn to the further work or information listed as desirable in sectons 4.3 and 4.15.

4. EVALUATION OF DATA FOR ACCEPTABLE DAILY INTAKE FOR MAN AND MAXIMUM RESIDUE LIMITS

EXPLANATION

This section contains brief comments on the compounds considered by the present meeting. The information provides a summary of the material that will appear in the monographs (pesticide residues in food - 1985), including details of further work or information considered necessary or desirable by the meeting. The requirements for further work or information are additional to those mentioned in earlier reports that have not been previously satisfied.

As in previous evaluations, compounds that were re-evaluated by the present meeting are marked with an asterisk. Compounds evaluated for the first time are identified by their chemical names, according to IUPAC nomenclature, as well as their common names. Standard common names of the International Organization for Standardization (ISO) are used wherever possible.

The estimated maximum acceptable daily intakes for man (ADIs) and maximum residue limits (MRLs), together with guideline levels (GLs) for some compounds with no currently estimated ADIs, appear also in Annex I. New MRLs classified according to commodity groups are listed in Annex II.A. Changes in MRLs are listed in Annex IIB.

In the case of some compounds, there will be no more detail in the 1985 evaluations than appears in this report (including its annexes). In other cases, an extended monograph or a monograph addendum will be included in the evaluations. A table, indicating the compounds on which a monograph containing additional information will appear, follows this explanation.

MONOGRAPHS

	Full Monograph		Monograph Addendum		No Monograph		Not considered	
	FAO	WHO	FAO	WHO	FAO	WHO	FAO	WHO
4.1 aldicarb			X			X		X
4.2 amitraz			X			X		X
4.3 azocyclotin					X	X	X	X
4.4 binapacryl			X	X				
4.5 bromomethane			X			X		X
4.6 bromophos			X			X		X
4.7 butocarboxim					X	X		
4.8 captafol			X			X		
4.9 carbendazim			X	X				
4.10 carbon disulphide			X			X		X
4.11 carbon tetrachloride			X			X		X
4.12 chlordimeform				X	X		X	
4.13 chlormequat			X			X		X
4.14 chlorothalonil			X	X				
4.15 cyhexatin					X	X		X
4.16 cypermethrin			X			X		X
4.17 2,4-D					X	X		X
4.18 deltamethrin			X			X		X
4.19 dialifos					X	X		X
4.20 dibromoethane			X			X		X
4.21 dichlofluanid			X			X		X
4.22 dichloroethane			X			X		X
4.23 diflubenzuron			X	X				
4.24 dimethipin	X	X						
4.25 dithiocarbamates			X			X		X
4.26 endosulfan					X	X		
4.27 ethephon			X			X		X
4.28 ethion					X	X	X	
4.29 fenamiphos				X	X		X	
4.30 fenvalerate					X	X		X
4.31 flucythrinate	X	X						
4.32 hexachlorobenzene			X			X		X
4.33 imazalil			X	X				
4.34 isofenphos					X	X		X
4.35 mecarbam			X			X		
4.36 metalaxyl			X			X		X
4.37 methamidophos				X	X		X	
4.38 methiocarb					X	X	X	
4.39 omethoate				X	X		X	
4.40 oxamyl			X	X				
4.41 paraquat					X	X	X	
4.42 permethrin			X			X		X
4.43 2-phenylphenol and its sodium salt			X	X				
4.44 phorate				X	X		X	
4.45 phosmet			X			X		X
4.46 phosphamidon					X	X	X	
4.47 pirimicarb			X			X		X

	Full Monograph		Monograph Addendum		No Monograph		Not considered	
	FAO	WHO	FAO	WHO	FAO	WHO	FAO	WHO
4.48 pirimicarb-methyl			X			X		X
4.49 prochloraz			X			X		X
4.50 propineb				X	X		X	
4.51 pyrazophos	X					X		
4.52 thiodicarb	X	X						
4.53 thiram					X	X		
4.54 triadimefon				X	X			
4.55 vamidothion			X	X				

4.1 ALDICARB*

Residue and analytical aspects

The meeting reviewed additional aldicarb supervised trials residue data for citrus and maize. In the case of citrus, additional residue data on lemons and Valencia oranges had been considered desirable to give added assurance that the 0.2 mg/kg limit was adequate. This added assurance was deemed highly desirable since the limit was based on a 90-day interval whereas 30 days is typical practice for some varieties.

The amount and type of citrus data provided were not as complete as was desirable. They were consistent with earlier JMPR conclusions that most aldicarb citrus residues from good agricultural practice would be below the current 0.2 mg/kg limit. However, some of the data give further evidence (from an additional country) that residues may reach or even exceed 0.3 mg/kg at short pre-harvest intervals. On the basis of available data the meeting confirmed the 0.2 mg/kg limit, but concluded that additional data on lemons at short pre-harvest intervals are still highly desirable.

The meeting had been requested by the CCPR to clarify limits for maize forage and fodder. The meeting noted that the 20 mg/kg maize forage limit (dry weight basis) was based on maximum residues of approximately 10 mg/kg (fresh weight basis) in several trials from one location. The meeting had recognized those trial data to be the possible result of contamination or analytical difficulties, but had no firm basis to discount them. New data from the same location and others allowed the meeting to conclude that disregarding data from three of the questionable trials could be supported, although the new data still show a tendency for higher residues from that location. Information was not sufficient to identify the reason, although moisture, temperature and soil type were likely factors. The meeting concluded that the new data, in conjunction with those previously submitted, would support a 5 mg/kg limit for maize forage on a fresh weight basis. The 0.05 mg /kg limit for maize grain and 2 mg/kg for maize fodder were confirmed.

The meeting reviewed additional data for aldicarb on potatoes, but did not have sufficient information to revise its 1979 recommendation of 1 mg/kg.

<u>Further work or information</u>

<u>Desirable</u> (from 1983 JMPR)

1. Additional good agricultural practice information, especially for potatoes, maize and sorghum.

2. Additional processing studies on maize and sorghum, with field-incurred residues at sufficiently high levels to allow a more conclusive estimate of residues in the various processed fractions.

3. Feeding studies on cattle at levels greater than 5 ppm in the diet.

4. Selected studies on lemons (and ideally also on Valencia oranges) in which aldicarb is applied in accordance with good agricultural practice at maximum recommended rates and harvested at approximately 30 days after treatment. Study details should be recorded, including the amount and frequency of precipitation or irrigation.

4.2 AMITRAZ*

<u>Residue and analytical aspects</u>

The meeting reviewed information submitted by The Netherlands on use patterns on animals and crops, on residue trials on cattle and on national residue limits. The information did not require any change in the existing recommendations.

4.3 AZOCYCLOTIN*

<u>Residue and analytical aspects</u>

See section 3.1.

<u>Further work or information</u>

<u>Desirable</u>

The availability of a method of residue analysis, suitable for regulatory purposes, which would distinguish residues arising from azocyclotin uses from those arising from cyhexatin uses.

4.4 BINAPACRYL*

<u>Toxicology</u>

The meeting reviewed the available toxicity data and concluded that the total data base is inadequate for establishing an ADI. At least, the following data will be required before the assessment of an ADI can be reconsidered:

1. Teratology study in rats.
2. Chronic toxicity/carcinogenicity studies in rats.
3. Carcinogenicity study in a second species.
4. Multi-generation reproduction study.
5. Pharmacokinetic studies.

6. Justification for the small doses administered in the rabbit teratology study.
7. In studies that were found to be invalid, possible neurological effects were noted. If these effects are observed in any of the above studies, they should be investigated further.

Residue and analytical aspects

In response to a request made by the CCPR at its 16th Session the meeting received information on approved and recommended uses of binapacryl in a substantial number of countries, but very little information was available on the actual extent of use of the compound.

Many supervised trials on apples have been carried out. Residues of binapacryl from these trials confirm the levels found in 1969. New trials were carried out on oranges, hops and cotton. In oranges residues were determined in the peel, pulp and juice and were present in all parts immediately after treatment, although mainly in the peel. The data on oranges and hops were adequate for the establishment of residue limits for these commodities.

Analytical methods have been developed using gas chromatography with electron-capture detection, and a method has also been published in which high-performance liquid chromatography is used for the final determination. It is possible to determine binapacryl by GLC without derivatization, and then to verify the presence of the compound after hydrolysis and methylation.

It should be noted that in the absence of an ADI the recorded levels are Guidelines Levels.

Further work or information

Desirable

1. Information on metabolism of binapacryl in crops and in soil.

2. Information on the actual extent of use of binapacryl.

4.5 BROMOMETHANE*

Residue and analytical aspects

The meeting reviewed information on current use patterns and limited data on residues in fruits in commerce and responded to a question from the CCPR. This information did not require any change in existing Guideline Levels.

4.6 BROMOPHOS*

Residue and analytical aspects

Additional information and residue data from The Netherlands confirmed that the MRLs of 0.5 mg/kg for pea straw and 2 mg/kg for carrots are appropriate.

4.7 BUTOCARBOXIM*

Toxicology

The toxicological data submitted to the present meeting were reviewed but could not be evaluated because of the lack of individual animal data in the reports of most of the studies.

A study of absorption, distribution, metabolism and excretion in rats, a rabbit teratology study, and a chronic toxicity and carcinogenicity study in a second rodent species with complete individual animal data will be needed before allocation of an ADI can be considered.

4.8 CAPTAFOL*

Toxicology

Captafol was assigned a temporary ADI in 1982 of 0-0.01 mg/kg body weight. Further studies required by 1985 included long-term oral studies in rats and mice. Two carcinogenicity studies in mice and a chronic toxicity study in rats were reviewed by the present meeting.

In one mouse study, captafol caused an increased incidence of haemangioendotheliomas of the heart and malignant tumours of the small intestine (Ito, et al., 1984). Incidences of haemangioendotheliomas were increased in a dose-related manner, and some metastasised. Incidences of both haemangioen-dotheliomas of the heart and of small intestine tumours were higher in male mice than in females. In the other mouse study (Eissenlord, and Wong, 1982), malignant tumours of the heart were observed in the high-dose group in both sexes and neoplastic lesions of the small intestine were observed in males, but in neither case were the increases statistically significant. Both studies therefore resulted in manifestation of similar biologically significant effects.

In the rat study (Cox et al., 1983), captafol caused an increased incidence of neoplastic lesions in the kidneys of males in the high-dose group which were also present in females at lower dose levels. Neoplastic nodules in the livers of females in the high-dose group were also significantly increased.

On the basis of the above studies, the meeting concluded that captafol is carcinogenic in both rats and mice. Because of the significance of the observed effect and because a no-effect level was not demonstrated, the temporary ADI was withdrawn.

The meeting considered it to be unnecessary to review other available data relating to the safety of captafol because of its conclusion regarding the carcinogenicity of the pesticide.

In view of the established carcinogenic potential of this compound, the meeting recommended that captafol should not be used where its residues in food can arise.

Residue and analytical aspects

The meeting reviewed some information on use patterns and some limited data on residues in potatoes. These did not require any changes in existing recommendations. However, the temporary ADI for captafol was withdrawn at this meeting and, in consequence, the meeting recommended that all temporary MRLs for this compound should also be withdrawn.

REFERENCES

Cox, R.H., Dudeck, L/E/, Tacey, R.L., Alsaker, R.D., Voelker, R.W., Dawkins,
        G., and Phipps, R.B.   (1983), Chronic Toxicity Study in Rats.
        DIFOLATAN.   Hazleton Laboratories.

Eissenlord, G.H. and Wong, Z.A. (1982), Lifetime Oncogenic Feeding Study of
        DIFOLATAN Technical (SX-945) in CD-1 (ICR-derived) Mice.
        Chevron Chemical Company, Ortho Division, Richmond, California.

Ito, N., Ogiso, T., Fukushima, S., Shibata, M., and Hagiwara, A. (1984),
        Carcinogenicity of Captafol in B6C3F$_1$ Mice, Gann. $\underline{75}$, 853-865.

4.9 CARBENDAZIM*

Toxicology

Carbendazim was last evaluated by the joint meeting of 1983 and an ADI was estimated to be 0-0.01 mg/kg bw using a 200-fold safety factor to reflect concern for the lack of individual animal data for many of the studies evaluated.

Additional data provided to the meeting alleviated some of the concerns regarding the reproduction and teratogenic studies on carbendazim. The NOEL of 2000 ppm was confirmed in the rat reproduction study. In separate rat and rabbit teratology studies additional individual animal data verified a NOEL for teratogenicity at 6000 ppm in both studies.

The meeting also recognized that there are valid long-term feeding studies and carcinogenicity studies for carbendazim which were utilized in the estimation of the ADI in 1983. However, substantial questions still remain concerning the absence of adequate macroscopic/microscopic records of the pathological examinations in separate rat carcinogenicity (Til et al., 1976), long-term dog (Reuzel et al., 1976) and mouse carcinogenicity (Beems et al., 1976) studies. In view of its continued concern over the lack of confirmatory laboratory data, the meeting was unable to consider increasing the existing ADI.

The meeting reaffirmed the desirability of the additional information identified by the 1983 JMPR.

Level causing no toxicological effect

Rat: 500 ppm in the diet, equivalent to 25 mg/kg bw.

Dog: 100 ppm in the diet, equivalent to 2.5 mg/kg bw.

Estimate of acceptable daily intake for man

0-0.01 mg/kg bw.

Residue and analytical aspects

The meeting reviewed some data on residues occurring in fruits and vegetables at points of retail sale in the United Kingdom. These did not require any changes in existing recommendations.

Further work or information

Desirable

1. Additional data/information are needed to clarify the apparent discrepancies between the macro- and microscopic findings in the long-term dog study and carcinogenicity studies in rats and mice identified in the 1983 and 1985 evaluations.

2. Additional information to elucidate the mechanism of degenerative testicular effects in mammals.

3. Elucidation of the variability of the mutagenicity data.

References

Beems, R.B., Til, H.P., and van der Heijden, C.A. (1976) Carcinogenicity study with carbendazim (99% MBC) in mice. Summary. Report No R4936 of the Central Institute for Nutrition and Food Research (TNO) submitted to WHO by BASF.

Reuzel, P.G.J., Hendriksen, C.F.M., and Til, H.P. (1976). Long-term (two-year) toxicity study with carbendazim in beagle dogs. Report from the Central Institute for Nutrition and Food Research (TNO) submitted to WHO by BASF.

Til, H.P., Köllen, C., and van der Heijden, C.A. (1976). Combined chronic toxicity and carcinogenicity study with carbendazim in rats. Report from the Central Institute for Nutrition and Food Research (TNO) submitted to WHO by BASF.

4.10 CARBON DISULPHIDE*

Residue and analytical aspects

The meeting reviewed some information concerning the occasional occurrence of carbon disulphide residues in cereals in commerce which did not require any change in existing Guideline Levels.

4.11 CARBON TETRACHLORIDE*

Residue and analytical aspects

The meeting reviewed some information on residues occurring in wheat in commerce which did not require any changes in existing Guideline Levels.

4.12 CHLORDIMEFORM*

Toxicology

Chlordimeform has been found to induce haemangiosarcomas in mice but not in rats (JMPR 1980). 4-Chloro-2-toluidine (previously termed 4-chloro-o-toluidine), a metabolite of chlordimeform, also produces haemangiosarcomas in mice but not in rats (IARC, 1983).

Data reviewed by the present meeting indicated that chlordimeform induced the activity of several hepatic drug-metabolising enzymes but the observed biological differences could not be attributed to the results of either _in vivo_ or _in vitro_ studies.

Studies of macromolecular binding of 4-chloro-2-toluidine to RNA and DNA of rat and mouse tissues _in vitro_ and _in vivo_ also could not explain the observed differences in response to this compound, nor could a study of its effect on the incorporation of ^{3}H-thymidine into capillary endothelial cells.

Chlordimeform was without mutagenic activity in various cellular systems but gave positive results in a cell transformation assay. The metabolites 4-chloro-2-toluidine and _N_-formyl-4-chloro-2-toluidine were positive in several reverse mutation assays but only with metabolic activation. The former metabolite was also positive in mouse lymphoma, cell transformation and DNA repair assays. Both produced chromosomal anomalies in at least one _in vivo_ assay.

Occupational studies indicate that haematuria and cystitis have occurred following incidents of relatively high exposure. Exposed workers readily absorb chlordimeform and the excretion of 4-chloro-2-toluidine can be monitored.

Data were submitted on the results of extensive urinary monitoring of chlordimeform applicators in seven countries. Results were variable but could not be adequately related to exposure, as information on the timing of exposure and sample collection was not provided. It is of interest to note that a daily excretion of 1.5 litres of urine containing 0.5 mg/l of 4-chloro-2-toluidine by a 60 kg individual approximates to absorption of 0.017 mg/kg body weight of chlordimeform.

Epidemiological data were not submitted.

The meeting was advised by the submitters of the data that chlordimeform is used only on cotton and that no other uses are anticipated. The meeting recommended that the use of chlordimeform be rigorously restricted to cotton production.

As the meeting considered that the available information partially met the requirement of the 1980 JMPR, it decided to extend the temporary ADI.

Level causing no toxicological effect

Rat: 2 ppm in the diet, equivalent to 0.1 mg/kg bw.

Dog: 250 ppm in the diet, equivalent to 6.25 mg/kg bw.

Estimate of temporary acceptable daily intake for man

0-0.0001 mg/kg bw.

Further work or information

Required (by 1987)

Interpretable epidemiological and urinary monitoring data on occupationally exposed workers.

Desirable

1.   Confirmatory long-term animal bioassay using a third species for evaluating the potential carcinogenic hazard.

2.   Further observations in man.

Reference

IARC (1983) IARC Monographs on the Evaluation of the Carcinogenic Risk of Chemicals to Humans, Vol. 30, pp. 61-72.

4.13 CHLORMEQUAT*

Residue and analytical aspects

Data suggesting that the limit for pears of 3 mg/kg estimated by the JMPR 1972 was too low for certain important pear cultivars were too limited to enable the meeting to estimate a higher figure.

4.14 CHLOROTHALONIL*

<u>Toxicology</u>

Chlorothalonil was evaluated by the joint meetings of 1974, 1977, 1979, 1981 and 1983 and additional metabolism data and a rat carcinogenicity study were requested.

These additional data provided to the 1985 joint meeting demonstrated preferential excretion via the bile and faeces, with secondary excretion in the urine. These metabolism data suggest metabolic pathways involving initial hepatic biotransformations, conjugation with reduced glutathione (GSH) and enzymic degradation. There is additional metabolism in the kidney, formation of thiol metabolites, and excretion in the urine. There was suggestion of additional metabolism in the kidney or the G.I. tract to a sulphur-containing, potentially nephrotoxic, compound. At higher doses there was a plateau of radioactivity in kidneys with subsequent slower removal. It was apparent that there is a shift in metabolism which occurs between doses of 50 and 160 mg/kg bw suggesting saturation of an active, rather than passive, uptake mechanism in the kidney.

Additional mutagenicity data submitted for rat and mouse bone marrow cytogenetic assays were negative. A hamster bone marrow cytogenetic assay was positive.

In 1983 the meeting expressed concern for the demonstrated nephrotoxicity and potential tumourigenicity which was evident from earlier studies in rats and mice. The mouse oncogenicity study reviewed in 1983 demonstrated compound-related effects on the kidney at and above 750 ppm, with a compound-related increased incidence of renal cortical tubular adenomas and carcinomas in males.

The rat oncogenicity study reviewed by this meeting demonstrated compound-related neoplastic changes in kidneys of treated males (at and above 800 ppm) and females (at and above 1600 ppm). Renal tubular adenomas and carcinomas were significantly increased in all dosed rats except low-dose females. There was also a decrease in time to tumour formation which was evident in the high-dose groups. Exposure of these rats to chlorothalonil in the diet produced a pronounced increase with dose in the occurrence and severity of renal tubular epithelial hyperplasia and chronic glomerulonephritis.

Chlorothalonil has also been evaluated by IARC (Vol. 30, 1983, IARC Monographs on the Evaluation of the Carcinogenic Risk of Chemicals to Humans). The evaluation determined that available oncogenicity data in rats and mice provided limited evidence of oncogenic potential to humans.

In 1974 the meeting evaluated five long-term studies in which rats were administered chlorothalonil at doses of 4 to 15,000 ppm with no evidence of a tumourigenic effect on the kidney, although there was clear evidence of epithelial degeneration and hyperplasia at doses above 60 ppm.

The meeting was informed of additional on-going oncogenicity studies in mice and rats, exposed via the diet to chlorothalonil. In consideration of these new studies, which are being conducted at lower doses than previous rat and mouse oncogenicity studies, the recognized change in metabolism at doses approximating 50 mg/kg bw, the absence of demonstrated mutagenic potential in

a complete battery of such assays, the absence of tumourigenic response in
several long-term studies reviewed in 1974, and the conflicting evidence from
carcinogenicity studies conducted by NCI, the meeting extended the TADI and
required the submission of these on-going tests when completed. However,
because of concern for the demonstrated oncogenicity in rodents the safety
factor used in estimating the temporary ADI was increased by the meeting.

<u>Level causing no toxicological effect</u>

Rat: 10 ppm in the diet, equivalent to 0.5 mg/kg bw.

Dog: 120 ppm in the diet, equivalent to 3 mg/kg bw.

<u>Estimate of temporary acceptable daily intake for man</u>

0-0.0005 mg/kg bw.

<u>Residue and analytical aspects</u>

The meeting evaluated additional information for chlorothalonil, which in
part was provided in response to earlier requirements. On the basis of
substantial new data the 1983 JMPR had concluded that the previously estimated
5 mg/kg limit for grapes might be exceeded, but needed additional information
for a firm conclusion. Although no new residue data were provided to this
meeting, additional required information on nationally approved uses gave
assurance that residue data already available (1979 and 1983 JMPR) reasonably
reflect good agricultural practice. Although data indicate that most residues
of chlorothalonil on grapes are likely to be no greater than the previously
estimated 5 mg/kg limit, levels exceeding 5 mg/kg from approved practices in
two widely separated geographical areas give sufficient reason to conclude
that the limit should be increased. A 10 mg/kg limit should be sufficient at
a common 7-day pre-harvest interval as opposed to the 46-day basis for the
current 5 mg/kg limit. This is the same as one national limit (where
supervised trials were conducted), less than the 25 mg/kg limit in one country
and more than the limit in other countries.

Additional supervised trials data for chlorothalonil on grapes from
additional countries are still desirable. Requirements for good agricultural
practice information on grapes have been met and the MRL remains temporary
only because the ADI is temporary. In view of the toxicological concerns
identified, the meeting emphasized that although residues arising from GAP on
grapes require an increase in the temporary MRL, this would not represent an
increased dietary exposure to chlorothalonil.

Additional information on supervised trials with chlorothalonil on
currants did not require a revision of the current limit, while data on
mushrooms were too few to support a limit. Only 4 of 163 samples of various
commodities (primarily small fruit) of unknown treatment history and sampled
at point of retail sale in the UK in 1981-1983 contained chlorothalonil
residues above 0.5 mg/kg. Residues in these four samples were well below the
Codex limits for the two commodities (currants and celery) which had such
limits.

<u>Further work or information</u>

<u>Required (by 1987)</u>

1. On-going carcinogenicity studies in rats and mice are understood to be in progress. Although the meeting recognized these studies are not scheduled for completion until September of 1988 and June of 1987, the meeting recommended any available data be submitted for evaluation when available.

2. Further metabolism data to identify the change in metabolic pattern with increasing dose, as well as further characterization of the GSH conjugation occurring in the G.I. tract and kidney.

<u>Desirable</u>

1. Supervised trials data on grapes from additional countries reflecting nationally approved uses.

2. Analyses of chlorothalonil-treated animal feed items (for example, bean and peanut vines), processed and unprocessed, for residues of PCBN (pentachlorobenzonitrile) (from the 1981 meeting).

3. Information on possible PCBN residues in tissues and milk of dairy cattle fed a diet containing chlorothalonil (from the 1981 meeting).

4.15 CYHEXATIN*

<u>Residue and analytical aspects</u>

See Section 3.1.

<u>Further work or information</u>

<u>Desirable</u>

The availability of a method of residue analysis, suitable for regulatory purposes, which would distinguish residues arising from azocyclotin uses from those arising from cyhexatin uses.

4.16 CYPERMETHRIN*

<u>Residue and analytical aspects</u>

The meeting reviewed information from The Netherlands on use patterns, and on residue trials on apples from The Netherlands and Sweden. The information did not require any change in existing recommendations.

Information was also received on national MRLs in The Netherlands.

The meeting also noted that the CCPR had replaced the proposed MRL for legume oilseeds by separate proposals for peanuts and soybeans at the same level (0.05** mg/kg). Since peanuts will, in future, be classified as an oilseed and since the level in peanuts is lower than the current recommendation for the group oilseed (0.2 mg/kg), the meeting proposed that this figure should now apply to the group in the classification "oilseeds except peanuts". The relevant recommendations would now be:

oilseeds except peanuts	0.2 mg/kg
peanuts	0.05** mg/kg
soybeans	0.05** mg/kg.

4.17 2,4-D*

<u>Residue and analytical aspects</u>

At the 16th Session of the CCPR several delegations requested information on the possible carry-over of 2,4-D from wheat and some other cereal grains arising from residues at harvest at the limit of 0.5 mg/kg, which was estimated by the 1980 JMPR.

This limit covers applications close to harvest which are occasionally necessary under certain climatic conditions.

Data were made available to the meeting on residues in wheat and flour arising from applications early in the growing season. In these trials levels of 2,4-D were very low or not measurable in the grain at harvest, and none was found in flour. The new data do not allow conclusions to be drawn on the possible carry-over into flour if the levels at harvest are of the order of 0.5 mg/kg.

4.18 DELTAMETHRIN*

<u>Residue and analytical aspects</u>

The meeting reviewed information submitted by The Netherlands on additional registered uses of deltamethrin in that country, together with some residues data from trials using deltamethrin to protect newly sown pasture and in the control of pests of dairy cattle. The meeting considered that the current uses of deltamethrin both directly on animals and on commodities used as animal feed justified an assessment of the possibility of residues being found in human foodstuffs of animal origin.

In response to a question from the 17th Session of the CCPR the meeting corrected an error in the report and evaluations of the 1980 JMPR concerning the estimated maximum residue level of deltamethrin in coffee beans. As a consequence, the MRL (a GL in 1980) is changed from 2 mg/kg to 0.02 mg/kg. There is no available information on the fate of deltamethrin residues in hops during the brewing process although carry-over of residues into beer would not be expected.

<u>Further work or information</u>

<u>Desirable</u>

1.   Data which could be used for the estimation of maximum residue levels of deltamethrin in food of animal origin.

2.   Information on the fate of deltamethrin residues in hops during the brewing process.

4.19 DIALIFOS*

Residue and analytical aspects

The CCPR at its 14th Session asked the JMPR to reconsider the definition
of the residue, currently "sum of dialifos and its oxygen analogue" for
commodities of plant origin and "dialifos" for commodities of animal origin.
Manufacture of dialifos has now ceased, and the 1982 JMPR withdrew the ADI.
The CCPR at its 17th Session agreed that the previously recommended MRLs
should be converted to GLs. The present meeting therefore considered the
definition of the residue.

Residue and analytical aspects of dialifos were evaluated in 1976. All
the residue data reviewed were for dialifos alone; there is therefore no
basis for including the oxygen analogue in the residue definition. It is
stated in the 1976 evaluations that dialifos <u>per se</u> is the residue of concern
on crops and that the oxon "has been detected at trace levels but was not
regarded as a significant component of the terminal residue". Analysis for
the oxygen analogue would in any case be unpractical since its limit of
determination is stated to be some ten times that of dialifos and it does not
survive the preferred regulatory clean-up procedures for dialifos.

It is concluded that the definition of the residue should be changed to
"dialifos" (for all commodities), the GLs remaining numerically unchanged.

4.20 1,2-DIBROMOETHANE*

Residue and analytical aspects

Information on current use patterns, fate of residues on cooking rice and
methods of residue analysis were reviewed by the meeting. This did not
require any changes in existing Guideline Levels.

4.21 DICHLOFLUANID*

Residue and analytical aspects

The meeting reviewed data from supervised trials on hops and grapes
provided to the 1985 JMPR by the manufacturers.

The new data on residues in hops showed a very large range of residues in
the limited number of trials. The meeting was unable to propose an MRL for
hops, dry.

In all four trials, beer prepared from hops harvested 14 days after the
last application and dried did not contain measurable amounts of dichlofluanid
(less than 0.1 mg/kg).

The new residue data on grapes confirm those evaluated at the earlier
meetings.

After reviewing all available data from supervised trials on cereal grains
it was recognized that insufficient data were available to support a group MRL
for cereal grains since data on residues from some main grain crops, such as
maize and rice, were lacking. The meeting, therefore, replaced the group MRL
for cereal grain commodities by estimates for the cereals for which data were
available, namely barley, oats, rye and wheat, all at the same level as the
group MRL, 0.1 mg/kg.

4.22 1,2-DICHLOROETHANE*

Residue and analytical aspects

Information on use patterns and an improved residue analysis procedure were reviewed by the meeting. The latter shows promise and its use should be encouraged. This information did not require any changes in existing Guideline Levels.

4.23 DIFLUBENZURON*

Toxicology

Diflubenzuron was reviewed by the 1981 JMPR and a temporary ADI of 0-0.004 mg/kg bw was estimated. Additional long-term feeding and carcinogenicity studies were required and these data have been evaluated by the 1985 meeting.

Dogs administered diflubenzuron orally for one year demonstrated effects consistent with met- and sulph-haemoglobinaemia at or above 10 mg/kg body weight, with a NOEL of 2 mg/kg body weight. These data demonstrate that the beagle dog is no more sensitive than the rat or mouse to the formation of met- and sulph-haemoglobin pigments from exposure to diflubenzuron.

Carcinogenicity studies in rats and mice were negative for oncogenic effects at 10,000 ppm. Non-neoplastic changes observed were consistent with those associated with met- and sulph-haemoglobin formation.

While the observation of measurable pathological changes (e.g. hepatocyte enlargement/vacuolation and haemosiderosis of the spleen and liver) was not evident except at higher dietary doses of diflubenzuron, the meeting nonetheless considered the elicitation of toxic methaemoglobinaemia to be the basis for estimating an ADI.

Level causing no toxicological effect

Rat: 40 ppm in the diet, equivalent to 2 mg/kg bw.

Mouse: 16 ppm in the diet, equivalent to 2.4 mg/kg bw.

Dog: 2 mg/kg bw/day.

Estimate of acceptable daily intake for man

0-0.02 mg/kg bw.

Residue and analytical aspects

Data providing information listed as desirable by the 1981 JMPR about the possible occurrence and content of the metabolite DFBA (2,6-difluorobenzoic acid) in milk, meat and eggs were made available.

From these data the meeting concluded that DFBA plays a minor metabolic role in cows, pigs, sheep and chickens. It was not identified in milk, and was a minor constituent in eggs. There is no need for further information on the possible occurrence of DFBA in milk, meat or eggs. The meeting confirmed that the residue limits should refer to diflubenzuron; DFBA should not be included in the residue definition.

Further work or information

Desirable:

Observations in man.

4.24 DIMETHIPIN
    2,3-dihydro-5,6-dimethyl-1,4-dithi-ine 1,1,4,4-tetraoxide

Dimethipin is a harvest-aid dessicant or moisture reduction chemical registered for use on oilseeds, potatoes and tomatoes. It was evaluated for the first time by the present meeting.

Toxicology

In rats, the compound is readily absorbed, metabolized and eliminated via the urine and faeces. It is degraded primarily to polar metabolites with less than 5% of a single oral dose being recovered as unchanged dimethipin in the excreta. In the goat, dimethipin is extensively degraded, also primarily to polar metabolites. Biotransformation of the compound includes hydrolysis, oxidation, decarboxylation, ring opening and conjugation.

Dimethipin has an oral LD_{50} value of about 500 mg/kg bw in mice and 1200 mg/kg bw in rats.

A two-generation (two litters/generation) reproduction study in rats as well as teratology studies in rats and rabbits were negative. Practically all of the mutagenic studies available were negative. The only positive mutagenic response was seen with the mouse lymphoma forward mutation assay and only in the presence of metabolic activation.

A one-year feeding study in dogs failed to show a no-effect level, mainly because of uncertainty concerning the presence of testicular degeneration even at 300 ppm, the lowest tested level. However, taking into consideration the lack of a dose-response relationship regarding incidence and severity of the testicular lesion, the absence of effect of the compound on the testis of rats in the two-generation reproduction study and the similarly negative effect in the testes of mice and rats in the long-term studies, plus the virtual absence of other toxic effects at the lowest tested level, it was concluded that a level somewhat below 300 ppm could reasonably be taken as a no-effect level for this species. In this connection, the meeting agreed that 100 ppm, the no-effect level established in an available 90-day dog feeding study, be accepted as a one-year no-effect level for this species.

In the long-term mouse and rat studies, there was seemingly an increase in incidence of lung adenocarcinoma in male mice of the top dosage group (2000 ppm) and of astrocytoma in male rats of both the intermediate and top dosage levels (i.e. 200 ppm and 1000 ppm). Although the evidence for a causal relationship between these particular tumour findings and treatment did not appear to be convincing, such a possibility could not be excluded at this time. Before a more definite opinion on the tumourigenic/carcinogenic potential of the compound can be expressed, additional information, as indicated under "Further work or information required" is needed on those mouse and rat studies from which data on historical control incidences of certain tumours (specifically lung tumours in mice and astrocytoma and liver tumours in rats) were obtained.

In view of the concerns with respect to increased incidence of lung adenocarcinoma in male mice and of astrocytoma in male rats of the long-term studies, a temporary ADI was estimated.

<u>Level causing no toxicological effect</u>

Mouse: 80 ppm in the diet, equal to 12.3 mg/kg bw.

Dog: 100 ppm in the diet, equivalent to 2.5 mg/kg bw.

<u>Estimate of temporary acceptable daily intake for man</u>

0-0.003 mg/kg bw.

<u>Residue and analytical aspects</u>

Data were sufficient for estimating limits as dimethipin <u>per se</u> in all crops under consideration except peas. Recommendations are listed in Annex I. In the case of grapes, no limits were recommended because dimethipin use on grapes is not GAP.

The fate of residues was investigated in plants, animals and soils, and during storage and processing. Dimethipin <u>per se</u> was the only compound identified in the plant studies, and it was 88.4, 20-25, 49, 48, and 14-97% of the total radioactivity in cottonseed, potatoes, rice grain, sunflower and grape juice, respectively. As many as 14 unidentified metabolites have been detected, the number depending on the crop.

Animal metabolism studies with ^{14}C ring-labelled dimethipin were conducted in rats, goats and chickens. Only 18 and 15% of the ^{14}C residues in goat liver and kidney respectively were identified with (butan-3-one-2-yl) 2-hydroxyethyl sulphone (III, due to ring cleavage) and 2,3,5,6-tetrahydro-5-hydroxy-5,6-dimethyl-1,4-dithi-ine 1,1,4,4-tetraoxide (IV) being the predominant residues. Only 2% of the ^{14}C residue was unchanged dimethipin. Unidentified residues included numerous polar metabolites and bound residues, part of which appeared to be glucuronide, cysteine and N-acetylcysteine conjugates. <u>In vitro</u> studies supported these as likely major metabolic steps. No information was provided as to whether total radioactivity was measured or residue identification attempted in muscle, fat or milk. In chicken liver and eggs 39% and 49% respectively of the ^{14}C residues were identified. Only 5.2% was identified in the kidney. While metabolites III and IV were the predominant residues in goat tissues, they were not significant residues in poultry tissues.

The chemicals 2-ethyl-2-methyl-1,3-dithiolane 1,1,3,3-tetraoxide (IX) and 2-(1-hydroxyethyl)-2-methyl-1,3-dithiolane 1,1,3,3-tetraoxide (X) were by far the major components in poultry tissues. It was thought that these resulted from IX being a component of the 2% of impurities in the labelled material. Unchanged dimethipin was a trace and 3.4% of the ^{14}C residues in liver and eggs respectively. With as much as 65-85% of the ^{14}C residues in tissues of animals unidentified and with no information on the amount (even as total radioactivity), characterization or identification of residues in muscle, fat or milk, it cannot be concluded that the fate of dimethipin in animals is well understood. No conventional feeding trials have been conducted.

Dimethipin residues in sunflower seed were shown to be stable up to 10 months in laboratory cold storage and up to three months in sunflower seed extracts stored at room temperature. Storage temperature was not stated for either.

In cottonseed processing studies, residues in hulls were as much as 36% greater than in the whole seed. Residues in meal were one third of those in the whole seed and residues in crude or refined oil and soapstock were significantly less than that. Results were similar in sunflower seed processing studies except that residues in hulls were frequently twice the level in the whole seed.

Analytical methods suitable for enforcement, which determine dimethipin _per se_ in plants and animal products, are available. The methods, by determining dimethipin _per se_, would normally be expected to determine approximately 10-90% of the total residue (dimethipin + metabolites) in plant products at harvest, depending on the commodity and interval after treatment. In animals however, only approximately 2% of the total residue would be determined by measuring dimethipin.

Further work or information

Required (by 1987)

1. Information on those mouse and rat studies from which data on historical control incidences of certain tumours, _viz_ lung tumours in CD-1 mice and astrocytoma and liver tumours in Sprague-Dawley rats, were obtained and presented in the submitted reports. (Information for each of the studies should include date of each study, age of animals at initiation, mortality rate of animals and experimental conditions such as diet, number of animals per cage, etc.)

2. Further pharmacokinetic and metabolic studies in rats and/or a non-rodent mammalian species using appropriate multiple dosage levels.

3. Acute oral toxicity studies on plant metabolites which are not found in mammals, if these are liable to occur as substantial residues.

4. Further identification or characterization of ruminant metabolites in liver, kidney, muscle, fat and milk, and of poultry metabolites in liver, muscle and fat. Depending on the results of these studies, conventional feeding studies and additional analytical methodology may be required before MRLs for animal products can be considered.

5. Determination as to whether metabolites detected in plants are the same as those identified in animals and soil.

6. Information on nationally approved uses for dimethipin on sunflower.

7. Results of soil metabolism studies reportedly recently completed.

Desirable

1. Results of diet analysis for the 18-month mouse and two-year rat feeding studies.

2. Studies on any potential oestrogenic or other hormonal effect of dimethipin including the determination of the affinity of the compound for steroid receptors.

3. Further studies in dogs to assess the effects, if any, of dimethipin on the testis.

4. Observations in man.

5. Additional residue data reflecting approved uses on commodities for which limits have been estimated.

6. Additional information on nationally approved uses.

7. Additional information on the fate of residues during storage and processing.

4.25 DITHIOCARBAMATE FUNGICIDES*

Residue and analytical aspects

The meeting was aware, on the basis of new data provided to the 1985 JMPR, that residues of ethylenebisdithiocarbamates (including residues from similar compounds such as thiram) on head lettuce often exceeded the limit of 1 mg/kg as carbon disulphide (CS_2) estimated by the JMPR in 1977.

This was especially the case if head lettuce was grown and harvested under glass or similar cover, under low temperature and low light conditions (late autumn and winter).

The new data enabled the meeting to estimate the higher maximum residue level of 5 mg/kg for head lettuce grown under these conditions.

The TMRL proposed is determined and expressed as mg CS_2/kg, and refers separately to the residues arising from any or each of the following groups of dithiocarbamates:

(a) dimethyldithiocarbamates

(b) ethylenebisdithiocarbamates, such as mancozeb, maneb, and zineb.

4.26 ENDOSULFAN*

Toxicology, residue and analytical aspects

The meeting discussed the present situation with regard to endosulfan and found it to be unsatisfactory. The meeting concluded that a complete re-evaluation is necessary. This should be based on current use patterns with toxicological data obtained following up-to-date protocols and residue data obtained using present analytical methods. The re-evaluation should also take into account the relevant information in the Environmental Health Criteria on endosulfan [1].

The required data should be submitted for study by the 1989 JMPR. Meanwhile, the absence of any indications of potential major adverse toxicological effects in man permits the extension of the TADI of 0.008 mg/kg bw.

---

[1]Endosulfan. Environmental Health Criteria 40. International Programme on Chemical Safety, World Health Organization, Geneva, Switzerland, 1984.

4.27 ETHEPHON*

Residue and analytical aspects

Information was received on a supervised trial on rye and on residues in fruit and vegetables in commerce. As only a little information has been received until now on residues from trials on cereals, the meeting was unable to recommend residue limits for ethephon in cereals.

Further work of information

Desirable

More information on approved uses and on residues from supervised trials on ethephon in cereals.

4.28 ETHION*

Toxicology

The required data for ethion were not made available to the 1985 JMPR, although the meeting was made aware of on-going studies needed for a decision on the temporary ADI. Because of the lack of support for maintaining the temporary ADI, the safety factor was doubled to provide a value of 0.0005 mg/kg bw. The meeting recommended that if the appropriate data are not submitted by 1986 the JMPR should consider withdrawing the temporary ADI.

Level causing no toxicological effect

Rat: 3 ppm in the diet, equivalent to 0.15 mg/kg bw.

Dog: 0.125 mg/kg bw/day.

Estimate of temporary acceptable daily intake for man

0-0.0005 mg/kg bw.

Further work or information

Required (by 1986)

1.   A short-term toxicity study in the dog.

2.   A teratology study in the rat.

3.   A reproduction study in the rat.

4.   A delayed neurotoxicity study.

5.   A long-term feeding study in the rat.

6.   A long-term oncogenicity study in a suitable species.

7.   Absorption, distribution and metabolism data in mammals.

Desirable

1.   Further observations in man

2.   Mutagenicity studies.

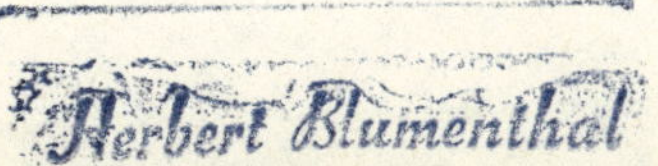

4.29 FENAMIPHOS*

<u>Toxicology</u>

Data evaluated by the 1985 meeting support the conclusions of the 1974 meeting with regard to acute toxicity and anti-cholinesterase potency. Various purities of technical fenamiphos (88 to 99.7 percent) produced the same degree of acute oral toxicity to rats. The major plant and animal metabolites were equally toxic.

Fenamiphos and its cholinesterase-inhibiting metabolites are better inhibitors of plasma than erythrocyte cholinesterase.

In a 100-day dog feeding study, fenamiphos inhibited only plasma cholinesterase in males at 1.7 ppm but not at 1.0 ppm.

Fenamiphos was not maternally toxic or teratogenic in rabbits at a dose of 0.1 mg/kg bw. However, fenamiphos was considered foetotoxic at all doses administered and to cause an increased incidence of chain fused sternebra at and above 0.3 mg/kg bw.

Fenamiphos was not oncogenic in a mouse carcinogenicity study, nor was it mutagenic.

Very limited new data were available which were evaluated and have been included in the monograph addendum. The meeting determined that additional studies, including rat oncogenicity, rat reproduction, rat teratology and rabbit teratology with a NOEL for foetotoxicity, are necessary for estimation of a full ADI.

A full re-evaluation was not performed but the meeting recommended that such an evaluation be performed when the on-going rat oncogenicity study becomes available in 1986. The existing ADI was changed to a temporary ADI which incorporated an increased safety factor to reflect the concern of the meeting about the foetotoxicity demonstrated in a rabbit teratology study.

<u>Level causing no toxicological effect</u>

Rat: 3 ppm in the diet, equivalent to 0.17 mg/kg bw.

Dog: 1 ppm in the diet, equivalent to 0.025 mg/kg bw.

<u>Estimate of temporary acceptable daily intake for man</u>

0-0.0003 mg/kg bw.

<u>Further work or information</u>

<u>Required (by 1987)</u>

1.   Submission of the results of on-going rat oncogenicity study.

2.   Submission of a full legible report and raw data for the rat teratology study.

3.   New rabbit teratology study to clarify the foetotoxicity observed at low dietary levels.

<u>Desirable</u>

Observations in man.

4.30 FENVALERATE*

<u>Residue and analytical aspects</u>

The meeting noted that the use of the new classification of foods and
animal feedstuffs (see para 2.7) for classifying oilseeds would result in a
withdrawal of the recommendation by the 1984 JMPR to combine the figures for
peanuts, 0.1 mg/kg, and soybeans, 0.1 mg/kg, in a single figure for legume
oilseeds of 0.1 mg/kg. The relevant recommendations would now revert to those
of the 1979 meeting, namely:

peanuts	0.1 mg/kg
soybeans	0.1 mg/kg.

The meeting considered the comment in the report of the 1985 CCPR
concerning paragraph 4.28 in the report of the 1984 JMPR.

The meeting noted that, although the 1984 JMPR had estimated a maximum
residue level of 0.1 mg/kg of fenvalerate likely to be found in milk in normal
agricultural practice, the recommendation was omitted. This omission is
corrected in the present report. Further consideration of the principles
involved in interpreting animal transfer studies in conjunction with realistic
estimates of the intake of pesticide residues by animals was postponed until
1986 (see also section 2.10).

4.31 FLUCYTHRINATE
   (<u>RS</u>)-α-cyano-3-phenoxybenzyl (S)-2-(4-difluoromethoxyphenyl)-3-
   methylbutyrate)

Flucythrinate is an insecticide related to the synthetic pyrethroids,
considered for the first time by the present meeting.

<u>Toxicology</u>

The principal mechanism of flucythrinate metabolism involves ester
cleavage and oxidation at the para-position of the alcohol moiety and at the
gem-dimethyl group of the acid moiety. Flucythrinate does not bioaccumulate
and the metabolites are mostly excreted in the urine and do not accumulate in
the tissues.

The toxicological profile of flucythrinate is similar to that of related
pyrethroids, although the acute oral toxicity is relatively high. The
production of hepatocellular tumours in the mouse is not considered to be of
biological significance, considering the known susceptibility of the mouse to
this effect.

Flucythrinate is not teratogenic in the rat or rabbit. The compound was
observed to cause mild maternal weight reduction in a reproduction study but
not at levels causing concern.

Flucythrinate has no dominant lethal effect in rats and was not mutagenic
in several assays.

<u>Level causing no toxicological effect</u>

Mouse: 30 ppm in the diet, equal to 4.0 mg/kg bw.

Rat: 30 ppm in the diet, equal to 1.6 mg/kg bw.

Dog: 100 ppm in the diet, equal to 2.5 mg/kg bw.

<u>Estimate of acceptable daily intake for man</u>

0-0.02 mg/kg bw.

<u>Residue and analytical aspects</u>

Flucythrinate is used against a wide range of noxious insects on many crops, including citrus, pome, stone and berry fruits, Brassicas, fruiting, leafy and root vegetables, cereal grains (pre-harvest), oilseeds, coffee and tea. It is registered or otherwise authorized in several countries around the world; more registrations are pending.

Flucythrinate is marketed in several formulations, including EC, WP and water-dispersible granules. Dosage rates are generally 25-75 g ai/ha (3-6 g ai/100 l).

Extensive information was provided on residues resulting from supervised trials in several areas of the world on various fruit crops and vegetables, cereal grains, including maize, some oilseeds, coffee, hops and tea.

The fate of residues in the meat of cattle, goats and poultry, milk of cattle and goats, and eggs was elucidated, and metabolites were identified. The fate of residues in soil and water, and during the processing or household preparation of treated commodities, such as apples (into sauce, pomace and cider), grapes (into juice and wine), hops and tea was also reported.

On most crops residues decline slowly. The decrease is in most cases far more dependent on growth between last application and harvest than on chemical breakdown of the residue. The residue is generally strongly absorbed onto the cuticle of the crop or to other surfaces, and hardly penetrates into the interior. Residues in the edible portions of crops of which the peel or pods are discarded (e.g. citrus pulp, peas and beans) are very low and generally not measurable. As a result of the low water solubility in combination with the strong absorption to organic material, there is negligible carry-over into the water phase during processing, e.g. from hops to beer, from grapes to wine and from manufactured dry tea to the infusion.

Various procedures for residue analysis have been developed. The method of choice is GLC with a ^{63}Ni electron-capture detector. The limit of determination is about 0.01-0.05 mg/kg. The method is suitable or can be adapted for regulatory purposes.

The available data enabled the meeting to estimate maximum residue levels on a number of crops, which are recommended as suitable for use as MRLs. They refer to flucythrinate alone.

<u>Further work or information</u>

<u>Required (by 1987)</u>

Information on residues in vegetable oils such as cottonseed oil and/or
other vegetable oils, crude and refined.

<u>Desirable</u>

1. Further studies on the biological activity of flucythrinate relevant
    to the mild nerve demyelination observed in the mouse and on possible
    effects on neurotransmitters.

2. Observations in man.

3. Additional information on residues from supervised trials on main
    crops on which flucythrinate is used, e.g. various citrus species,
    leafy vegetables such as lettuce, including glasshouse lettuce,
    fruiting vegetables including glasshouse crops, legume vegetables
    (pods and seeds).

4. Information on actual residues found in meat, fat, milk and eggs
    after feeding treated animal feed crops or other crops of which
    wastes are used as animal feeds, e.g. straws of cereal grains, vines
    and/or straws of legume vegetables, etc.

4.32 HEXACHLOROBENZENE*

<u>Residue and analytical aspects</u>

At the 16th Session of the CCPR (1984) the Committee agreed that there was
a need to review the Guideline Levels for hexachlorobenzene (HCB) in the light
of residue data from recent monitoring programmes. The CCPR requested the
JMPR to review any information received and to consider estimating ERLs for
food commodities including those for which no levels had been estimated
previously.

In response to the request from the Codex Secretariat to provide relevant
data to the JMPR, only five countries provided data on the current position
with respect to the occurrence of HCB residues in food in their countries.

Although the data show a tendency to decreased HCB residue levels in
several food commodities in recent years, they are still too scanty to allow a
full review of the existing Guideline Levels or the estimation of ERLs for
other commodities.

<u>Further work or information</u>

<u>Desirable</u>

Recent data on HCB residues in food and feed commodities of animal and
plant origin from monitoring programmes in various regions of the world;
these data should preferably not be more than three to four years old.

4.33 IMAZALIL*

Toxicology

Previous meetings have recognized the need for an adequate long-term evaluation in rats. The data submitted were considered sufficient to determine a NOEL of 100 ppm for non-oncogenic effects. There was no evidence of oncogenic potential at dietary levels up to and including 400 ppm. Short-term mutagenicity tests were negative.

Although one teratology study was evaluated, the meeting was aware of several other teratology studies which have not been presented in full to the JMPR. Considering its desire to review these data, the meeting recommended continuation of the temporary ADI at the same level.

Level causing no toxicological effect

Rat: 100 ppm in the diet, equal to 5 mg/kg bw.

Dog: 1.25 mg/kg bw/day.

Estimate of temporary acceptable daily intake for man

0-0.01 mg/kg bw.

Residue and analytical aspects

Additional residue data submitted to the 1985 JMPR by the manufacturer supported the current temporary MRLs for pome fruits, potatoes, strawberries and tomatoes. The meeting also examined residue data from post-harvest treatments on peaches, nectarines and plums, from which it was able to estimate a maximum residue level for stone fruits of 5 mg/kg.

Further work or information

Required (by 1986)

Additional teratology studies known to be available but which have not been submitted to the JMPR.

Desirable

Observations in man concerning the use of certain imidazole compounds, such as anti-fungal drugs.

4.34 ISOFENPHOS*

Residue and analytical aspects

At the request of the CCPR, the meeting reviewed the data on residues in maize fodder and sweet corn fodder reported in the 1981 evaluations. It recognized that residues of isophenfos plus its oxygen analogue in these commodities could occasionally exceed 0.2 mg/kg and confirmed its previous estimate of 0.5 mg/kg as a maximum residue level in these commodities.

4.35 MECARBAM*

Toxicology

The required data for mecarbam were not made available to the 1985 JMPR, although the meeting was made aware of ongoing studies needed for a decision on the temporary ADI. Because of the lack of support for maintaining the temporary ADI, the safety factor was doubled to provide a value of 0.0005 mg/kg bw. The meeting recommended that if the appropriate data are not submitted by 1986 the JMPR should consider withdrawing the temporary ADI.

Level causing no toxicological effect

Rat: 5 ppm in the diet, equivalent to 0.21 mg/kg bw.

Dog: 5 ppm in the diet, equivalent to 0.15 mg/kg bw.

Estimate of temporary acceptable daily intake for man

0-0.0005 mg/kg bw.

Residue and analytical aspects

The meeting examined information provided by Spain on GAP of mecarbam, and extensive residue data from supervised trials on citrus fruit carried out in four Spanish provinces, which included data on the mandarin group (satsumas and clementines), oranges and lemons. These data supported the current temporary MRL on citrus fruit of 2 mg/kg for a pre-harvest interval of 14 days.

Further work or information

Required (by 1986)

1.   An adequate delayed neurotoxicity study in hens.

2.   Full report on the metabolic studies in rats.

3.   Complete metabolic studies in laboratory animals other than the rat.

4.   A ruminant metabolism study.

5.   Should the ruminant metabolism study indicate any possibility of residues of concern in animal tissues or milk other than those identified in plants, data should be provided on those residues occurring in meat and milk from feeding ruminants with a diet containing residues found in treated citrus.

Desirable

1.   Observations in man.

2.   Additional information on nationally registered or approved uses on additional commodities (especially olives, olive oil, fruits and vegetables) and supervised trials data reflecting those uses.

4.36 METALAXYL*

Residue and analytical aspects

The meeting reviewed information on some current use patterns and data on residues from supervised trials on a range of additional fruit and vegetable crops; residue data on citrus fruit and on grapes following a change in use pattern were studied. Some data from residue monitoring studies on lettuce on retail sale was also reviewed. Information on an improved method of residue analysis which determines the total residue of metalaxyl and its metabolites which contain the 2,6-dimethylaniline moiety was also available. A question from the CCPR on the limit of determination on avocado was answered. The information available allowed the meeting to suggest levels that were suitable for the establishment of MRLs for metalaxyl on apples, Brussels sprouts, cottonseed, pineapples, soybeans and strawberries and amended values on grapes and avocados. (see Annex 1).

Further work or information

Required (by 1986)

In line with the comments made at the 17th Session of the CCPR (Report para. 160), the meeting concluded that a full re-evaluation of the residue data on all appropriate crops should be carried out using data based on the use of the improved analytical method which determines the total residue of metalaxyl together with its metabolites which contain the 2,6-dimethylaniline moiety.

4.37 METHAMIDOPHOS*

Toxicology

Methamidophos was re-evaluated in 1982, when a temporary ADI was estimated. Long-term and carcinogenicity studies in rats and a reproduction study in mammals were required.

Additional pharmacokinetic and metabolism studies indicate that methamidophos is rapidly absorbed, distributed, metabolized and excreted, mainly via urine as acid metabolites and through the expired air as CO_2.

In addition to the rabbit study evaluated in 1982, a no-effect level for embryotoxic/teratogenic effects was established in a rat study. A no-effect level was also found from data for reproductive effects.

Methamidophos was found to be non-mutagenic in bacterial and _in vivo_ assays. There were no indications of oncogenicity in a mouse oncogenicity study or in a rat chronic toxicity/oncogenicity study. A new one-year dog study confirms the NOEL used for the derivation of the 1982 temporary ADI.

Methamidophos caused delayed polyneuropathy in man following excessive exposure. However, maximum tolerated doses in hens failed to cause delayed neuropathy.

The toxicology monograph prepared by the present meeting supersedes the monograph prepared in 1976.

<u>Level causing no toxicological effect</u>

Rat: 2 ppm in the diet, equivalent to 0.1 mg/kg bw.

Dog: 2 ppm in the diet, equal to 0.06 mg/kg bw.

<u>Estimate of acceptable daily intake for man</u>

0-0.0006 mg/kg bw.

<u>Further work or information</u>

<u>Desirable</u>

Observations in man.

4.38 METHIOCARB*

<u>Toxicology</u>

An ADI of 0-0.001 mg/kg bw was estimated for methiocarb in 1981. The 1983 JMPR recommended that further work was desirable to clarify the plasma cholinesterase inhibition observed in the dog study, which provided the NOEL for establishing the ADI.

The present meeting reviewed several new studies, including a two-year feeding study in mice, which provided additional data on cholinesterase inhibition. The detailed data in the dog study previously requested were not submitted.

The meeting concluded that the primary concern with the use of methiocarb, following application as a bird repellent to consumer crops, was that its residues may exceed the NOEL, resulting in acute toxic effects in humans. The meeting agreed to leave the existing ADI unchanged at 0-0.001 mg/kg bw.

The meeting confirmed the views expressed by the 1983 JMPR and the recommendation that the relevant MRLs should be withdrawn.

4.39 OMETHOATE*

<u>Toxicology</u>

A temporary ADI for omethoate was estimated in 1971. The toxicology of the compound was reviewed by the JMPR in 1975, 1978, 1979 and 1981, at which time a carcinogenicity study in a rodent species at higher dose levels was required, while further mutagenicity studies were desirable.

The results of an adequate chronic toxicity/oncogenicity study in mice, in which neither oncogenic effects nor other somatic damage were observed, were provided to the meeting.

A no-effect level of 1.0 mg/kg bw was determined for embryotoxic/teratogenic effects in the rabbit.

Delayed neuropathy was not observed in hens. No potential for delayed neuropathy was observed in man.

Omethoate was found mutagenic only in gene conversion and mitotic recombination tests in <u>S. Cerevisiae</u> D7, whereas other tests were negative.

The meeting estimated an ADI for omethoate.

<u>Level causing no toxicological effect</u>

Rat: 1 ppm in the diet, equivalent to 0.05 mg/kg bw.

Dog: 0.025 mg/kg bw/day.

<u>Estimate of acceptable daily intake for man</u>

0-0.0003 mg/kg bw.

<u>Further work or information</u>

<u>Desirable</u>

Observations in man.

4.40 OXAMYL*

<u>Toxicology</u>

Oxamyl was evaluated by the Joint Meeting in 1980 and 1984, and a full ADI was estimated. Data concerning the dimethylcyanoformamide (DMCF) metabolite, inadvertently omitted from the 1984 monographs, were evaluated by the 1985 meeting.

Data presented on the DMCF metabolite demonstrated moderate acute oral toxicity in rats, a negative response in a mutagenicity assay and a NOEL of 50 ppm in a 90-day rat feeding study.

These data do not alter previous evaluations for oxamyl and the ADI for oxamyl was reaffirmed.

<u>Level causing no toxicological effect</u>

Rat: 50 ppm in the diet, equivalent to 2.5 mg/kg bw.

Dog: 100 ppm in the diet, equivalent to 2.5 mg/kg bw.

<u>Estimate of acceptable daily intake for man</u>

0-0.03 mg/kg bw.

<u>Residue and analytical aspects</u>

The meeting reviewed additional supervised trial data and good agricultural practice (GAP) information submitted in response to requirements previously listed by the JMPR and to questions raised at the CCPR. Additional data or GAP information were required on some commodities before reconsideration of the temporary MRL status. It has also been questioned whether some uses which were the basis of MRL estimates are in fact good agricultural practice. The meeting also considered questions on the definition of the residues referred to it by the CCPR.

The meeting determined that, except for kidney bean (dry), all GAP and residue data requirements have been met to allow all temporary MRLs to be changed to MRLs. For kidney beans (dry), confirmation of nationally approved uses is necessary before the temporary status is removed.

On the basis of GAP and available residue data, estimated MRLs were confirmed for kidney beans (dry), apples, tomatoes, cucurbits (except cucumbers) and potatoes. In the case of root and tuber vegetables a group limit is recommended to replace the equivalent level for individual members of this group. In the case of citrus and celery, GAP was confirmed and existing data supported MRL increases to 5 mg/kg for each. The meeting recommended an MRL of 2 mg/kg for cucumbers, on the basis of the available data.

From the available data, the meeting revised several limits to reflect maximum residue levels expected when oxamyl is used in practice and when the reported interval between last application and harvest is observed. The levels refer to the sum of oxamyl and its oxime, expressed as oxamyl, and are listed in Annex 1.

The meeting concluded that the previously requested feeding study on pigs is no longer needed and that the general requirement for residue data on animal feed items has been met.

The meeting concluded that available information does not indicate a need to include the DMCF (dimethylcyanoformamide) metabolite in the definition of the residue for enforcement purposes, although it recognized that an analytically significant proportion of the total residue in plants may be DMCF.

<u>Further work or information</u>

<u>Required (by 1986)</u>

Evidence of nationally approved uses for oxamyl on kidney beans, dry.

<u>Desirable</u>

1. Observations in man.

2. Additional residue data from supervised trials reflecting good agricultural practice in additional countries, in particular, residue data for peas (from 1983 JMPR).

3. Information on residues in foods in commerce and at consumption (from 1983 JMPR).

4. Information on the effects of cooking, processing, and storage on oxamyl residues in raw agricultural commodities (from 1983 JMPR).

5. Crop rotation studies on additional commodities and under field conditions with applications of commercial formulations (both granular and liquid) according to maximum recommended application rates (from 1983 JMPR).

4.41 PARAQUAT*

Toxicology

Paraquat was last evaluated by the 1982 JMPR, at which time a temporary ADI of 0-0.001 mg;kg bw (as paraquat dichloride) or 0-0.0007 mg;kg bw (as paraquat ion) was estimated. The 1982 meeting requested additional data by 1985 from a chronic toxicity/carcinogenicity study in the rat, a 12-month oral study in the dog, and a multigeneration study in the rat.

Data were submitted to the present meeting that met the 1982 JMPR request (Ashby, R. et al. (1983) "Paraquat: Combined Toxicity and Carcinogenicity Study in Rats", unpublished report from Life Science Research Laboratory submitted to the World Health Organization by Imperial Chemical Industries PLC; Ishmael, J. and Godley, M.J. (1983) "Paraquat: Lifetime Feeding Study in Rats: Histopathological Examination of Lungs", unpublished report from ICI Central Toxicology Laboratory submitted to the World Health Organization by Imperial Chemical Industries PLC; Kalinowski, A.E. et al. (1983) "Paraquat: One-year Feeding Studies in Dogs", unpublished report from ICI Central Toxicology Laboratory submitted to the World health Organization by Imperial Chemical Industries PLC; Lindsay, S. et al (1982) "Paraquat: Multigeneration Reproduction Study in Rats - Three Generations", unpublished report from ICI Central Laboratory submitted to the World Health Organization by Imperial Chemical Industries PLC).

These data were reviewed, but logistical difficulties precluded their full evaluation, especially in light of the considerable amount of information previously evaluated by the JMPR. The meeting therefore recommended that a complete evaluation of all valid data available on paraquat should be undertaken by the 1986 JMPR.

The meeting was aware that the two-year study in rats had been considered by one national authority to indicate a possible oncogenic potential in the rat. In examining these data, differing interpretations of the observed lesions by different pathologists were apparent to the meeting. Further, the meeting was aware of the divergent response in the target organ (lung) which appears to exist between the rat and man.

In considering these factors, the meeting did not feel that sufficient concern existed to warrant withdrawing the TADI, which is therefore extended until 1986. Meanwhile, the data on historical evidence, and full descriptions of lesions of the lung, in the strain of rat utilized in the study of concern, in the testing laboratory are required.

Level causing no toxicological effect

Rat: 30 ppm in the diet, equivalent to 1.5 mg/kg bw.

Estimate of temporary acceptable daily intake for man

0-0.001 mg/kg bw as paraquat dichloride (0-0.0007 mg/kg bw expressed as paraquat ion)

Further work or information

Required (by 1986)

1.   Submission of all data available for complete re-evaluation.

2.   A submission of historical control data on all lung lesions.

4.42 PERMETHRIN*

Residue and analytical aspects

The meeting reviewed information on the use pattern of permethrin on lettuce in The Netherlands, the reported rates of application being appreciably lower than those reported in 1982. Trials data from the use of permethrin on tomatoes in New Zealand did not require any change in recommendations. Monitoring data from the United Kingdom on over 200 samples of apples, peas, cucumbers and tomatoes demonstrated residues in only 12 samples, all well below the relevant MRLs.

In accordance with the request from The CCPR (ALINORM 85/24A, para 180), the meeting considered the relationship between the MRL of 1 mg/kg in the carcase fat of meat of cattle, pigs and sheep and the MRL of 0.1 mg/kg in milk.

Although 0.1 mg/kg had been estimated as a maximum residue that could occur in milk from treated animals (1980 Evaluations, p. 370), bulk milk in trade is unlikely ever to reach such a level.

The meeting noted that the level found in the fat of milk was not necessarily identical with the level in carcase fat. It is not valid to draw conclusions from the comparison of a determined value in carcase fat with one calculated for fat of milk from residue levels in whole milk.

4.43 2-PHENYLPHENOL AND ITS SODIUM SALT*

Toxicology

The toxicology of 2-phenylphenol (OPP) and its sodium salt (SOPP) was previously reviewed by the JMPR in 1962, 1969 and 1983. Just prior to the 1983 meeting, new information consisting of biochemical, teratogenic, carcinogenic and mutagenic data became available and was evaluated at the meeting. A final working paper which reviewed the recently submitted data was not completed, however, at that time. The present working paper reviews the data previously submitted in 1983 together with additional information submitted in 1985. It should be noted that nearly all of the data reviewed in this working paper is from the published literature or from unpublished reports originally submitted to the JMPR by member countries. Reports of studies generally did not contain the detailed information ordinarily present in reports submitted by the pesticide industry. Nevertheless, information presented in these reports is considered sufficient to support the statements and conclusions presented in this working paper.

In 1983, the JMPR agreed that OPP and SOPP should be considered as equivalent for the purposes of toxicological evaluation and should be dealt with together since the use of SOPP results in OPP residues in agricultural commodities. Furthermore, SOPP was established as a bladder carcinogen in the rat. Although fewer data on OPP were available, a similar pattern of neoplastic response in rats was noted. The existing ADI for OPP and SOPP was converted to a temporary ADI and the safety factor was simultaneously increased from 100 to 5000 to reflect the concerns of the meeting. In addition, further information to permit adequate evaluation in the future was required to be submitted to the JMPR by 1985. The additional toxicological information included:

1.   information on the progress of a multigeneration reproduction study,

2.   information on the progress of a carcinogenicity/chronic toxicity study in a rat strain known to be sensitive to induction of bladder carcinomas (a strain other than Fischer F344),

3.   metabolic, pharmacokinetic and other related studies, as appropriate, in the strains of animals tested in long-term studies for carcinogenicity,

4.   additional metabolic and pharmacokinetic studies in other species and strains of animals.

In response to the requirement for further information, a protocol for a proposed two-generation reproduction study in rats using OPP as the test material has been received. No information on the progress of a new carcinogenicity/chronic toxicity in rats has been received. Some new metabolic and pharmacokinetic data have been received but they are very limited with respect to elucidating possible biochemical mechanisms of action of carcinogenicity.

An IARC monograph on OPP and SOPP was published in 1983. This document summarized chemical and physical data, production, use and occurrence of these chemicals. It also evaluated biological data relevant to the oncogenic risk to humans that was available prior to 1983[1].

Recent carcinogenicity studies on sodium 2-phenylphenate (SOPP) have reported statistically significant increased incidences of carcinomas in the urinary bladder, and some in the renal pelvis, of male F344 rats following administration of 1% and 2% SOPP in the diet. In female F344 rats, an increased, but lower, incidence of urinary bladder neoplasms was also reported at a dietary dosage level of 1%. Similar tumours observed at lower dietary dosage levels (0.5% and 0.7%) in male and female rats, although not statistically significant, were considered to be biologically relevant owing to the rarity of these tumours in this rat strain and their absence in control animals. There does not appear to be a cause-effect relationship between stones and neoplasms in the urinary bladders of rats. SOPP has been determined to be a carcinogen to the urothelium of F344 rats.

Although fewer carcinogenicity studies on 2-phenylphenol (OPP) are available, some recent evidence suggests that OPP may also be a carcinogen on the urinary bladder of male F344 rats at dietary dosage levels of 1.25% and 2.5%. Another earlier study did not, however, demonstrate a similar response in male or female Wistar rats. OPP has not been adequately tested to permit any conclusion as to carcinogenicity to be finalized.

Carcinogenicity studies in mice with both OPP and SOPP were negative for tumourigenic effects. The dosage level in the OPP study may have been too low to permit expression of tumours.

---

[1]   International Agency for Research on Cancer (1983) IARC Monographs on the Evaluation of the Carcinogenic Risk of Chemicals to Humans, Miscellaneous Pesticides, 30: 329-344.

Mutagenicity assays with OPP and SOPP in bacteria have been overwhelmingly negative, although weakly positive results have been occasionally noted in isolated instances. Results of studies in cultured mammalian cells have been mixed. Both negative and weakly positive responses in several assays have been reported. Results from _in vivo_ studies have been regularly negative.

A series of _in vitro_ and _in vivo_ biochemical studies suggested the possibility that an altered metabolic pathway for OPP/SOPP, occurring at high dosage levels only, may be related to (and presumably responsible for) the occurrence of urothelial tumours at similar dosage levels in long-term studies. Although this speculation appears plausible at this time, considerably more direct experimental support will be required before it can be accepted as fact.

Teratology studies on rats using OPP as the test material were negative for teratogenic effects.

With respect to the oncogenic potential of OPP and SOPP, the meeting compared results from available oncogenic studies to the low anticipated dietary exposures to OPP and SOPP. On the basis of this comparison and other information, the meeting agreed to extend the temporary ADI for OPP/SOPP to 1989.

Level causing no toxicological effect

Rat: 2000 ppm in the diet, equivalent to 100 mg/kg bw.

Dog: 500 mg/kg bw/day.

Estimate of temporary acceptable daily intake for man

0-0.02 mg/kg bw.

Residue and analytical aspects

2-Phenylphenol was evaluated by the meeting in 1969, 1975 and 1983. The main use of 2-phenylphenol and its sodium salt is as a post-harvest fungicide on fruits and some vegetables, with most being used on citrus fruits intended for the fresh fruit market.

Information reviewed by the meeting included current use patterns and recent extensive residue data from supervised trials on citrus fruit, with limited data on other fruits. The bulk of the residue remains on the peel of citrus fruit, only low microgramme quantities being detected in the edible portions of treated fruits. Very little is extracted from the peel by tea or alcohol. Data from monitoring studies of food in commerce confirmed the trials data. Total diet studies in Japan and the USA confirm that actual dietary intakes are very much lower than any estimates based on MRLs or residue values for whole fruits might suggest.

Improved methods of residue analysis were reported which should be suitable for regulatory purposes.

The information available to the meeting fully supported the current recommendations in regard to maximum residue levels for 2-phenylphenol. No changes or additions are required.

<u>Further work or information</u>

<u>Required (by 1989 or earlier)</u>

1.   A multigeneration reproduction study.

2.   A carcinogenicity/chronic toxicity study in a rat strain known to be
      sensitive to induction of bladder carcinomas (a strain other than
      Fischer F344).

3.   Metabolic, pharmacokinetic and other related studies, as appropriate,
      in the strains of animals tested in long-term studies for
      carcinogenicity and in other species, including a consideration of
      species, sex and dosage level differences.

4.   Qualitative and quantitative monitoring data on the urinary excretion
      of OPP and/or its metabolites by industrial workers, or others,
      regularly exposed to OPP or SOPP.

5.   Mutagenicity studies on urinary metabolites of OPP and/or SOPP.

<u>Desirable</u>

Additional observations in man.

4.44 PHORATE*

<u>Toxicology</u>

The toxicology of phorate was considered by the meeting in 1977, 1982 and
1983. Owing to the lack of an appropriate delayed neurotoxicity study, only a
temporary ADI was allocated in 1982. In 1983, the required study was not
available. The meeting extended the temporary ADI, however, to 1985. The
required neurotoxicity study and additional mutagenicity studies were
submitted for evaluation in 1985.

Phorate did not induce clinical or histopathological signs of
neurotoxicity in a study in hens. No evidence of mutagenic potential was
observed in a series of mutagenicity studies.

Since all required toxicity studies have been submitted and evaluated, the
meeting estimated an ADI for phorate.

<u>Level causing no toxicological effect</u>

Rat: 1 ppm in the diet, equivalent to 0.05 mg/kg bw.

Dog: 0.01 mg/kg bw/day.

<u>Estimate of acceptable daily intake for man</u>

0-0.0002 mg/kg bw.

<u>Further work or information</u>

<u>Desirable</u>

Observations in man.

4.45 PHOSMET*

Residue and analytical aspects

The meeting reviewed information submitted by The Netherlands on an additional use on cattle, some residues data on milk from a trial use of phosmet on cattle and their national MRLs. The information did not require any change in existing recommendations.

4.46 PHOSPHAMIDON*

Toxicology

The required data for phosphamidon were not made available to the 1985 JMPR, although the meeting was made aware of ongoing studies needed for a decision on the temporary ADI. Because of the lack of support for maintaining the temporary ADI, the safety factor was doubled to provide a value of 0.0005 mg/kg body weight. The meeting recommended that if the appropriate data are not submitted by 1986 the JMPR should consider withdrawing the temporary ADI.

Level causing no toxicological effect

Rat: 2 ppm in the diet, equivalent to 0.1 mg/kg bw.

Dog: 0.5 mg/kg bw/day.

Estimate of temporary acceptable daily intake for man

0-0.0005 mg/kg bw.

Further work or information

Required (by 1986)

1.   The following replacement or new studies:

    (a)   two-year rat study
    (b)   12-month dog study
    (c)   two-generation reproduction study in rats
    (d)   teratology studies in rats and rabbits
    (e)   mutagenicity studies

2.   An appropriate delayed neurotoxicity study

Desirable

Further studies on the metabolites of phosphamidon and their toxicities.

4.47 PIRIMICARB*

Residue and analytical aspects

Additional residues data from Spain supported the MRL of 0.5 mg/kg for oranges, recommended by the 1981 meeting on the basis of data from Portugal.

<u>Further work or information</u>

<u>Desirable</u>

Additional data on residues in citrus fruit from countries where applications close to harvest are permitted, and on residues in citrus varieties of smaller size.

4.48 PIRIMIPHOS-METHYL*

<u>Residue and analytical aspects</u>

In response to requests made at previous meetings, information on current use patterns and residue data from supervised trials on peanuts and from revised use patterns on citrus were received and reviewed. Data from supervised trials on dried fish were also received.

Current use patterns on citrus fruits lead to higher residue levels than those reviewed earlier and a level of 2 mg/kg is required to cover this situation, as compared with the level of 0.5 mg/kg previously recommended. This would still generally lead to less than 0.05 mg/kg in the flesh of treated fruit.

Extensive data on residues in peanuts and their products indicated that the MRLs reported at the 1976 meeting, which were based on limited information, were somewhat high for whole peanuts (50 mg/kg) and peanut kernels (5 mg/kg); the current data supported MRLs of 25 mg/kg and 2 mg/kg respectively. On the other hand, the MRL for peanut oil (10 mg/kg) is too low to cover current expected residue levels.

The data on residues in dried fish were adequate for the estimation of a maximum residue level of 10 mg/kg.

4.49 PROCHLORAZ*

<u>Residue and analytical aspects</u>

The fungicide prochloraz was first evaluated by the 1983 joint meeting which estimated maximum residue levels or temporary limits for several commodities. Estimates for cereals, mushrooms and citrus fruit were for prochloraz only, while estimates for tropical fruits and rapeseed were for total residues of prochloraz and metabolites hydrolyzable to the 2,4,6-trichlorophenol moiety. Estimates for the commodities expressed as total residues were temporary pending receipt of sufficient information to permit an estimate on the basis of prochloraz <u>per se</u>. All estimates for fruit were also **temporary pending receipt of information** on **nationally** approved uses. Other requirements, including ruminant and poultry metabolism studies, needed to be met before estimates for residues in animal products were possible, and other information was considered desirable.

On the basis of new studies the meeting concluded that the relation between free prochloraz and total residues was either not determinable or highly variable on these commodities, depending on the commodity and type of treatment. Because of this and other information, the meeting agreed that all MRLs should be expressed as total residues. Accordingly, new estimates in terms of total residues were made for cereals. New estimates were unnecessary for mushrooms and citrus, where residue levels have been shown to be similar whether expressed as prochloraz or total residues.

Requirements for approved use information have been met for banana, avocado and mango, for which new data were consistent with previous estimates. New residue data also supported previous estimates for citrus, stone fruit and rapeseed. New or additional data were insufficient to support estimates for strawberries, sugarbeet, eggplant, pepper, potatoes or lettuce. Although fairly substantial data on peas and tomatoes were available, the meeting decided not to estimate limits since not even proposed use information was available.

None of the required metabolism studies have yet been provided for poultry. Results of a single-dose cow metabolism study and a 28-day calf feeding study were available. The metabolism study indicates that 85% of bovine liver and kidney residues were composed of three hydroxy metabolites plus BTS-44770 and BTS-3037 (free). Together the three hydroxy metabolites may account for approximately 40% of liver and kidney residues. Residues in other tissues or milk were not identified or characterized. The meeting concluded that the metabolism is sufficiently understood for temporary limits in animal products. Other information is needed for full MRLs.

Information was provided on the effects of processing on residues in mushrooms in response to the request of the 1983 JMPR. Data indicate that residues in dehydrated mushrooms are 3-4 times greater than in fresh, apparently the result of water loss since in absolute terms there is a decrease in residues. Residues were less in preserved mushrooms than in fresh; no comparison could be made for canned mushrooms.

The 1983 JMPR required an analytical method suitable for enforcement purposes for animal products before consideration could be given to MRL estimates for animal products. Such a method was provided to this meeting and is similar to analytical methods previously reviewed by the JMPR, which determine residues hydrolyzable to 2,4,6-trichlorophenol. The procedure would be expected to determine approximately 60-90% of total animal residues.

In response to questions from the 1983 JMPR on the possibility of interference in the total residue procedures by other pesticides containing the 2,4,6-trichlorophenol moiety, the meeting was given assurances that this was unlikely to occur.

Maximum residue level estimates are listed in Annex 1.

<u>Further work or information</u>

<u>Required (by 1987)</u>

1.   Information on nationally approved uses for citrus, stone fruits and papaya.

2.   Poultry metabolism study.

3.   A conventional feeding trial in poultry.

4.   A conventional feeding trial on a lactating ruminant, with the feeding of compounds representative of residues expected from field trials on crops at recommended and exaggerated rates.

<u>Desirable</u>

1. Quantification of individual residues of BTS-54906, BTS-54907,
    BTS-54908, BTS-44770 and free BTS-3037 identified in liver and kidney
    in the cow metabolism study.

2. A ruminant metabolism study continued for at least three days at
    sufficiently high dosage to permit identification of residues in milk
    and tissues in addition to liver and kidney.

3. Documentation that the analytical procedures separate
    2,4,6-trichlorophenol from other trichlorophenols.

4. Validation of the analytical method for animal products utilizing the
    major trichlorophenol animal metabolites BTS-44770 and BTS-3037.

4.50 PROPINEB*

<u>Toxicology</u>

The toxicology of propineb was previously reviewed by the meeting in 1977,
1980 and 1983. Because of concern of the meeting in 1977 regarding the
potential for thyrotoxicity and tumourigenicity of propylenethiourea (PTU), a
breakdown product of propineb, the meeting estimated only a temporary ADI for
man. Although no new toxicity data were provided in 1980, the meeting took
into account available data on ethylenethiourea (ETU), an analogous breakdown
product of the ethylenebisdithiocarbamates. Further evaluation of propineb
was postponed pending the submission of additional data. After examining the
available data in 1983, the meeting concluded that a complete evaluation was
not possible. Adequate data for evaluation were required to be submitted by
1985. Meanwhile, the temporary ADI was extended until then. Data submitted
for evaluation in 1985 consisted of long-term mouse and rat studies,
mutagenicity studies and a special study on the effect of PTU on DNA. In
addition, data previously submitted for evaluation in 1983 were re-examined.
These data included several studies on propineb (acute toxicity studies,
short-term study on thyroid function in rats, mutagenicity studies and an
oncogenicity study on mice) and on PTU (pharmacokinetic studies on rats and a
long-term thyroid function study on rats).

An oncogenic study on mice with propineb indicated increased hepatocellular adenomas in male mice and increased pulmonary adenomas in female mice
at 800 ppm in the diet, the highest dosage level tested. These increases in
tumours may have been related to administration of the test material. Thyroid
tumours were not induced in treated mice in this study. A NOEL for
non-neoplastic effects could not be determined in this study, however, owing
to insufficient data.

In a long-term study on mice with PTU, an increased incidence of hepatocellular adenomas was observed in male mice at 1000 ppm in the diet, the
highest dosage level tested. Increased incidences of hepatocellular carcinomas were also observed in male mice at 10 ppm and higher. In the same
study, increased incidences of hepatocellular adenomas and carcinomas were
observed in female mice at 100 ppm and higher. Thyroid tumours attributable
to PTU were not observed, but increased thyroid hypercellularity was noted in
male mice at 1000 ppm.

In long-term rat studies with propineb, previously reviewed by the JMPR,
an increased incidence of thyroid benign tumours was observed at 1000 ppm and

higher in the diet. Non-neoplastic thyroid effects were observed in the same study at 100 ppm and higher. In another study, increased liver and kidney weights were observed at 100 ppm and higher. A NOEL of 10 ppm was determined. In a long-term study on rats with PTU, thyroid tumours were not related to treatment with PTU except at 1000 ppm in the diet, which was a clearly excessive dosage level. Goitrogenic effects in the thyroid were observed, however, at dosage levels as low as 1 ppm, the lowest dosage level tested. A NOEL could not be determined in this study.

Short-term studies on thyroid function in rats with propineb did not establish an unequivocal NOEL for effects on the thyroid. In a long-term study on thyroid function in rats with PTU, effects on the thyroid were observed at 1000 ppm in the diet. Ambiguous effects were observed at lower dosage levels. Pharmacokinetic studies on rats with PTU demonstrated preferential uptake of radioactivity from ^{14}C-labelled PTU by the thyroid.

Mutagenic studies on propineb and PTU were negative or inconclusive. A special study on the effect of PTU on DNA demonstrated increased DNA synthesis in mouse spleen cells. PTU did not bind to the DNA of mouse liver cells.

In view of the carcinogenic response in the liver of mice to PTU and the lack of a NOEL for thyroid effects of propineb in a long-term study in mice in short-term studies in rats and for PTU in a long-term study in rats, the meeting recommended that the temporary ADI for propineb be withdrawn.

In view of the established carcinogenic potential of this compound, the meeting recommended that propineb should not be used where its residues in food can arise.

<u>Residue and analytical aspects</u>

In view of the withdrawal of the temporary ADI for propineb and the toxicological findings concerning PTU, the meeting agreed to withdraw previously estimated TMRLs for propineb and Guideline Levels for PTU.

4.51 PYRAZOPHOS
    ethyl 2-diethoxyphosphinothioyloxy-5-methylpyrazolo[1,5-<u>a</u>]pyrim=
    idine-6-carboxylate

Pyrazophos is a systemic pesticide especially active against powdery mildews. It is formulated as wettable powder and emulsifiable concentrate, both containing 30% active ingredient. It is mainly used on cereals, apples, strawberries, cucurbits and hops.

Pyrazophos has not been reviewed previously by the meeting.

<u>Toxicology</u>

The data base submitted in support of this compound did not include sufficient details to permit the estimation of an ADI. Before the assessment of an ADI can be reconsidered, all the data relating to the safety of pyrazophos, including detailed data on all aspects of individual animals, should be submitted.

<u>Residues and analytical aspects</u>

Metabolic studies have been carried out on and in plants, in cattle and in soils. Disappearance from leaf and fruit surfaces is mainly caused by evaporation. Residues on cucumbers 14 days after treatment consisted mainly of the parent compound, but metabolism or degradation on leaves from wheat plants was more extensive. In wheat plants residues 19 days after application consisted of 19% parent compound and 81% metabolites. The main metabolite is 2-hydroxy-5-methyl-6-ethoxycarbonylpyrazolo[1,5-a]pyrimidine, presumably as a β-glucoside conjugate. In one experiment a compound was observed which behaved as the oxygen analogue of pyrazophos on TLC.

Residues of pyrazophos in muscle, fat and milk from a lactating cow 26 hours after intake were low, while residues in kidney and liver were 0.72 and 0.24 mg/kg. The half-life of pyrazophos in two different standard soils was 30-40 days.

Residues of pyrazophos and pyrazophos oxon in plants, animals and soil can be determined by gas chromatography with a flame photometric detector.

<u>Further work or information</u>

<u>Required (by 1987)</u>

Information on residues in meat and milk from cattle fed a diet containing pyrazophos.

<u>Desirable</u>

1.   Information on residues in meat from pigs and meat and eggs from poultry fed a diet containing pyrazophos.

2.   Additional information on the identities and quantities of metabolites in plants after treatment with pyrazophos.

3.   Information on the effect of processing on residues in crops.

4.52 THIODICARB
3,7,9,13-tetramethyl-5,11-dioxa-2,8,14-trithia-4,7,9,12-tetra-azapentadeca-3,12-diene-6,10-dione

Thiodicarb is a non-systemic carbamate insecticide with a relatively narrow spectrum of activity closely related to its first metabolite methomyl. It is specific against Lepidopterous pests, controlling larvae at different stages as well as eggs in many instances.

Thiodicarb was reviewed for the first time by the JMPR in 1985.

<u>Toxicology</u>

Thiodicarb is rapidly absorbed, metabolized and excreted, and has not been demonstrated to accumulate in animal tissues. It is degraded to methomyl, which is converted to the "oxime" (methyl hydroxythioacetimidate) and ultimately to acetonitrile, carbon dioxide, acetic acid and acetamide. The ultimate metabolic fate in animals depends on the isomeric configuration of methomyl (<u>Z</u> or <u>E</u>).

The acute oral toxicity (LD_{50}) in rats is 66-120 mg/kg, depending on the vehicle used. In monkeys an acute oral LD_{50} is 467 mg/kg bw.

Thiodicarb causes reversible cholinesterase inhibition. Long-term feeding and oncogenicity studies in rats and mice have revealed no oncogenic potential

in either species and a NOEL of 3 mg/kg for non-oncogenic effects was
determined. No adverse reproduction or teratogenic effects in rats or mice
have been demonstrated.

Thiodicarb was not mutagenic in a wide variety of assays. However, it was
positive in the mitotic gene conversion assay using <u>Sacharomyces cerevisiae</u>.

In two short-term feeding studies in dogs, thiodicarb demonstrated adverse
liver effects in 90 days at doses at or above 15 mg/kg bw, while in a
six-month study at doses up to 45 mg/kg no adverse effects were observed at 15
mg/kg body weight. Considering the conflicting information concerning liver
effects in dogs, the meeting required the submission of an on-going one-year
dog study by 1987. A temporary ADI was therefore estimated.

<u>Level causing no toxicological effect</u>

Rat: 60 ppm in the diet, equivalent to 3 mg/kg bw.

<u>Estimate of temporary acceptable daily intake for man</u>

0-0.01 mg/kg bw.

<u>Residue and analytical aspects</u>

Thiodicarb formulations are registered in 17 countries and are used mainly
on cotton, grapes, maize, soybeans, tobacco and tomatoes. The recommended
rates and pre-harvest intervals for some of these crops are as follows: On
cotton, rates from 0.4 to 1.0 kg ai/ha per treatment applied as many times as
needed, with a PHI of 28 days. On soybeans, rates from 0.50 to 0.84 kg ai/ha
per treatment applied as many times as needed, with a PHI of 28 days. On
field corn, rates from 0.55 to 1.10 kg ai/ha applied as many times as needed
but not exceeding a total of 4.5 kg ai/ha per season with a PHI of 28 days.
On sweet corn, rates from 0.56 to 0.84 kg ai/ha applied as many times as
needed at intervals between 1 and 7 days but not exceeding a total of 8.4 kg
ai/ha per season and with a PHI of 0 days. On tomatoes, rates from 0.45 to
1.1 kg ai/ha applied as many times as needed with a PHI of 0 days.

Sufficient residue data and information on corresponding good agricultural
practices were available for cotton, soybean, field corn, sweet corn and
tomatoes and consequently the meeting could recommend TMRLs for these crops.

The fate of thiodicarb has been studied in animals, plants and soil. In
animals the metabolic pathway of thiodicarb involves cleavage to methomyl,
oxidation of the latter to methomyl sulphoxide, hydroxylation of the <u>N</u>-methyl
group of methomyl and hydrolysis to the methomyl "oxime" methyl hydroxythioacetimidate and its sulphoxide. Conjugation of the three latter
metabolites results in the formation of water-soluble glycones. Other
metabolic reactions result in the formation of CO_2 and acetonitrile as the
major end-products. In laying hens no residues of thiodicarb or methomyl <u>per
se</u> were found in poultry tissues or eggs. In lactating cows the results were
similar and no carbamate residues were found in any of the milk samples or
body tissues.

In plants the metabolic pathway is very similar. A considerable amount of
radioactivity was lost as volatile compounds, carbon dioxide and acetonitrile. The organosoluble metabolites consisted of two major components,
thiodicarb and methomyl, one minor component, the "oxime" and three minor
unidentified metabolites. From the water soluble metabolites, at least seven

aglycones were obtained, two minor aglycones, methomyl and the "oxime", and five major components (naturally occurring products formed by incorporation of radiolabelled carbon dioxide). Little or no absorption and translocation of thiodicarb occurred from the treated leaves, indicating the non-systemic nature of the compound.

In sandy loam soil the half life of thiodicarb was about 30 days.

Analytical methods for thiodicarb residues have been developed by the manufacturer and validated for many crops. Extraction with a mixture of 9:1 acetone: water or acetone:methanol is followed by a coagulation procedure to remove interfering co-extractives. Caustic hydrolysis converts thiodicarb and methomyl to "methomyl oxime". The total residue is then extracted from the acidified aqueous sample with dichloromethane. After clean-up and dissolution in acetone, the sample is analyzed by gas chromatography using a flame photometric detector equipped with a filter specific for sulphur.

Thiodicarb residues consist essentially of thiodicarb and its degradation product methomyl. "Methomyl oxime" is also quantitated by the method of analysis, but is not a significant residue.

Further work or information

Required (by 1987)

1. Submission of on-going one-year dog feeding study known to be in progress.

2. Information on possible effect on maternal body weight gain demonstrated in a rat teratology study.

Desirable

1. Observations in man, including monitoring of acetamide in urine.

2. Analytical method for the parent compound.

3. Feeding study on milking cattle with treated crops.

4.53 THIRAM*

Toxicology

Thiram has had a temporary ADI since 1967. The compound was last reviewed by the 1980 JMPR, at which time data relating to a full evaluation of the teratogenic potential of thiram and studies to resolve its effects, including thiram-induced anaemia, which were reported to the 1977 JMPR in summary form only, were requested by 1983. These data were not submitted for consideration by the 1983 JMPR, so the temporary ADI was extended to 1985.

New data relating to these effects were not submitted to the present meeting. The temporary ADI for thiram was therefore withdrawn.

The meeting was not aware of any new concerns caused by residues of thiram; however, the total data base is inadequate for establishing an ADI. The assessment of all the data relating to the safety of thiram will be required before the estimation of an ADI can be reconsidered.

<u>Residue and analytical aspects</u>

As the temporary ADI for thiram was withdrawn by the meeting, in the absence of the further toxicological data required, the meeting agreed that the MRLs previously estimated for thiram should be converted to Guideline Levels.

4.54 TRIADIMEFON*

<u>Toxicology</u>

A temporary ADI was estimated for triadimefon by the 1983 JMPR. That meeting required clarification of the toxicological significance of hepatic toxicity in rats and mice and of the hyperplastic liver nodules observed in chronic mouse feeding studies.

In chronic feeding studies in the mouse, rat and dog, triadimefon produced a dose-related increase in liver weight accompanied by elevation of serum hepatic alkaline phosphatase and transaminase activities. The rat was most sensitive but enzymatic induction was readily reversible on cessation of exposure. The mouse was the only species tested which exhibited significant histopathological changes with hyperplastic liver nodules but only at the highest dose level tested, 1800 ppm (JMPR, 1981).

In feeding studies, triadimefon increased the liver weights of dogs, rats and mice which, in dogs and mice, correlated with biochemical evidence of hepatotoxicity at higher doses. Reversible induction of hepatic microsomal enzymes of rats and mice also occurred. It is known that induction of hepatic microsomal activity can be accompanied by compensatory hepatic hyptertrophy. These related effects were fully reversible in the rat, the species found to be most susceptible to microsomal enzyme induction.

Previous <u>in vitro</u> studies have shown that triadimefon binds to hepatic cytochrome P-450, and is a modest inhibitor of microsomal enzyme activities. Further studies show that rat liver homogenate reduces triadimefon to the corresponding alcohol, triadimenol, and that triadimefon does not adversely affect DNA, as indicated by the Pol test with <u>E. coli.</u>

The 1984 JMPR considered the toxicological significance of hepatic tumours in the mouse, including those associated with the administration of high doses of pesticides able to induce hepatic microsomal enzymes. Viewed in that light, the present meeting considered that the toxicological significance of the hyperplastic liver nodules observed in chronic mouse feeding studies with triadimefon was adequately clarified.

The meeting was therefore able to estimate an ADI of 0.03 mg/kg bw.

<u>Level causing no toxicological effect</u>

Mouse: 300 ppm in the diet, equivalent to 40 mg/kg bw.

Rat: 50 ppm in the diet, equivalent to 2.5 mg/kg bw.

Dog: 230 ppm in the diet, equivalent to 8.25 mg/kg bw.

<u>Estimate of acceptable daily intake for man</u>

0-0.03 mg/kg bw.

<u>Residue and analytical aspects</u>

Temporary MRLs for triadimefon have been recommended for several commodities, and the limits refer to the sum of triadimefon and its main metabolite triadimenol.

At the 17th Session of the CCPR, the JMPR was requested to re-examine the residue definition for the following reasons:

1.   There were indications that there were residues on some plants for which there were no metabolic studies.

2.   Conjugated residues were not determined, although methods were now available which would determine free and conjugated residues in plants and animals.

3.   The most recent feeding trials data examined by the JMPR (1983) were based on these more recent methods.

The meeting has considered these observations. The evaluations of 1979, 1981 and 1983 mentioned the presence in plants of metabolites other than triadimenol, namely 4-chlorophenol, an oxidation product of triadimefon and a mixture of the glycosides of triadimenol, 4-chlorophenol and the oxidation product. In some experiments where cereals were treated with ^{14}C-triadimefon, the levels of these metabolites were determined.

In some feeding trials (1983 evaluations), total residues were determined in the milk and tissues of cattle and in poultry and eggs. In all other supervised trials and feeding trials, only residues of triadimefon and triadimenol were determined.

The meeting concluded that the definition of the residues should continue to refer only to the sum of triadimefon and its main metabolite triadimenol. The reason for this was that a change of the definition to include some of the minor metabolites would require new data for all supervised trials on plants. Furthermore, it was proposed by the 1983 JMPR that limits should be expressed in terms of a single compound whenever possible. However this is not appropriate for triadimefon, since the main metabolite, triadimenol, has similar fungicidal uses and therefore should be included in the definition.

<u>Further work of information</u>

<u>Desirable</u>

Observations in man.

4.55 VAMIDOTHION*

<u>Toxicology</u>

Vamidothion was evaluated in 1973 and 1982, at which time a temporary ADI was estimated.

Several studies, including a teratogenicity study, a multigeneration reproduction study, a delayed neurotoxicity study, and a dog study of adequate duration were required in 1982.

The teratogenicity (rat, rabbit) studies gave no indication of vamidothion
having embryotoxic/teratogenic potential at dose levels up to 20 mg/kg bw/day.

Vamidothion was not mutagenic in some bacterial systems, while in some
others it was positive only at very high concentration levels. Vamidothion
induced a low SCE and chromosomal aberration _in vitro_ but in an _in vivo_
micronucleus test no conclusion could be reached because of the small number
of animals used.

No delayed neuropathy was induced in hens.

Pending the receipt of a one-year dog study and a multigeneration
reproduction study, the meeting decided to maintain the temporary ADI at the
level set in 1982.

Level causing no toxicological effect

Mouse: 1 ppm in the diet, equal to 0.137 mg/kg bw.

Rat: 1 ppm in the diet, equal to 0.054 mg/kg bw.

Dog: 5 ppm in the diet, equivalent to 0.125 mg/kg bw.

Estimate of temporary acceptable daily intake for man

0-0.0003 mg/kg bw.

Residue and analytical aspects

Vamidothion was evaluated by the JMPR in 1973 and 1982. At the latter
meeting a temporary ADI was estimated and the Guideline Levels recorded in
1973 were converted to temporary MRLs.

The present meeting received new information on the current use patterns
of vamidothion, including currently recommended dosage rates and pre-harvest
intervals.

Information was also provided on residues from supervised trials on some
additional crops and from countries not included in the 1973 evaluations.

The use of vamidothion on Brussels sprouts is no longer recommended. The
TMRL arising from the GL recorded for this commodity in 1973, without
supporting data from supervised trials, should therefore now be withdrawn.

The new data on grapes confirm those recorded in 1973. The data on citrus
fruits and raspberries, in both cases from only one country, are insufficient
to estimate maximum residue levels.

The analytical method of choice, which can be used or adapted for
regulatory purposes, is GLC with a ^{63}Ni electron-capture detector. Limits
of determination are 0.02-0.05 mg/kg.

On the basis of the new data, together with those evaluated in 1973, the
meeting estimated the maximum residue levels listed in Annex I which are
recommended as being suitable for establishing TMRLs. The limits are for the
sum of vamidothion, its sulphoxide and its sulphone, expressed as vamidothion.

<u>Further work or information</u>

<u>Required (by 1988)</u>

1.   Multigeneration reproduction study.

2.   One-year dog study.

<u>Desirable</u>

Observations in man.

5.   RECOMMENDATIONS

5.1   In the interests of public health and agriculture and in view of the
needs of the Codex Committee on Pesticide Residues, the meeting
<u>recommends</u> that Joint Meetings on Pesticide Residues should continue
to be held annually.

<u>RECOMMENDATIONS FROM SECTION 2.</u>

5.2   The meeting <u>recommends</u> that the current mode of distribution of JMPR
reports and evaluations be examined, and where appropriate revised,
in order to ensure their receipt by all relevant ministries and
their availability to interested institutions and individuals. This
revision should also be undertaken with the aim of increasing the
visibility of the work of the JMPR.

5.3   The meeting noted that an international meeting to update the
principles and methodology governing the assessment of the
toxicology of pesticide residues in food will be organized in the
near future. The present meeting <u>recommends</u> that this
international meeting be requested to   consider the toxicological
basis and data requirements for the estimation of an ADI or
temporary ADI, and to provide general guidance on relevant
toxicological methodology.

5.4   The meeting <u>recommends</u> that efforts be made to increase the general
awareness of the work of the JMPR and to improve understanding of
the ways in which MRLs and ADIs can be used in a scientifically
acceptable manner.

5.5   The meeting <u>supports a recommendation</u> in the discussion paper,
"Codex Limits for Pesticide Residues in Food and Consumer Safety",
prepared by a CCPR Working Group, that a special joint FAO/WHO
meeting should be convened to develop guidance for those seeking
assurance that adherence to maximum residue limits in individual
commodities contributes to ensuring the safety of food to consumers.

5.6   The meeting <u>recommends</u> that the procedures outlined in the discussion
paper (see 5.5 above), using the concepts of theoretical daily intake
(TDI) and estimated daily intake (EDI) to estimate potential dietary
exposure to pesticide residues, should be explored together with
other relevant procedures which could contribute to a better
appreciation of the issues involved. The meeting <u>also recommends</u>
that it is essential that this matter be considered in full detail
by the next JMPR.

5.7   Because some of the oncogenicity studies in mice reviewed by the
meeting did not include haematology determinations, the meeting
<u>recommends</u> that haematology determinations in future oncogenicity
studies in mice should be performed at least at termination.

<u>RECOMMENDATIONS FROM SECTION 4</u>

5.8   As a consequence of the withdrawal of the temporary ADIs for
captafol and propineb at this meeting, the meeting <u>recommends</u> that
all temporary MRLs for captafol and propineb and guideline levels
for propylenethiourea (PTU) should be withdrawn. The meeting <u>further</u>
<u>recommends</u> that neither captafol nor propineb should be used where
their residues in food can arise.

5.9   The meeting <u>recommends</u> that the use of clordimeform be rigorously
restricted to cotton production.

5.10   The meeting <u>recommends</u> that if the appropriate data for ethion,
mecarbam and phosphamidon are not submitted by 1986, the JMPR should
consider withdrawing the temporary ADIs.

5.11   In the light of the toxicological evaluation at this meeting, the
meeting <u>confirms the recommendation</u> of the 1983 JMPR that the MRLs
for methiocarb in apples, blueberries, cherries, currants (red),
grapes and peaches should be withdrawn.

6. <u>FUTURE WORK</u>

The following items should be considered at the 1986 and/or 1987 meeting.

1. Pesticides scheduled at the present or at a previous meeting for re-
evaluation in 1986/1987. These include:

1.1 For toxicological evaluation:

1.1.1 1986:

from 1982 meeting - isofenphos, methacrifos, triazophos;
from 1984 meeting - carbosulfan, chlordane, fenitrothion, fenvalerate,
                    propamocarb;
from 1985 meeting - ethion, imazalil, mecarbam, phosphamidon.

1.1.2 1987:

from 1983 meeting - bitertanol;
from 1984 meeting - acephate, dimethoate, methiocarb;
from 1985 meeting - chlordimeform, chlorothalonil, dimethipin,
                    fenamiphos, thiodicarb.

1.2 For residue evaluation:

1.2.1 1986:

from 1983 meeting - fenitrothion;
from 1984 meeting - bitertanol, cyhalothrin, diflubenzuron;

from 1985 meeting - metalaxyl, oxamyl.

1.2.2. 1987:

from 1984 meeting - carbosulfan, methoprene;
from 1985 meeting - chlorothalonil, dimethipin, flucythrinate,
                      prochloraz, pyrazophos.

2. Pesticides recommended for priority attention by the 17th (1985) Session
    of the CCPR:

    2.1 For toxicological evaluation:

        2.1.1 1986:

        glyphosate, vinclozolin.

        2.1.2 1987:

        benalaxyl, cyfluthrin, fluvalinate, propiconazole.

    2.2 For residue evaluation

        2.2.2 1986:

        benalaxyl, cyfluthrin, fluvalinate, glyphosate, propiconazole,
        vinclozolin.

3. Pesticides listed for evaluation in 1985 or previous meetings, but not
    considered fully for various reasons:

    3.1 For toxicological evaluation:

        3.1.1 1986:

        clofentezine, methomyl, paraquat.

        3.1.2 1987:

        coumaphos, chinomethionat, ethoprophos, folpet, permethrin.

    3.2 For residue evaluation:

        3.2.1 1986:

        clofentezine, dinocap.

4. Reconsideration of MRLs, ADIs and Assessment of Consumer Risk
    (Recommendation of the 1985 JMPR).

7. <u>REFERENCES</u>

PREVIOUS FAO AND WHO DOCUMENTS

FAO/WHO.
1962
Principles governing consumer safety in relation to pesticide resi-
dues. Report of a meeting of a WHO Expert Committee on Pesticide
Residues held jointly with the FAO Panel of Experts on the Use of
Pesticides in Agriculture. FAO Plant Production and Protection
Division Report. No.PL:1961/11: WHO Technical Report Series,
No. 240.

FAO/WHO.
1964
Evaluation of the toxicity of pesticide residues in food; report of
a Joint Meeting of the FAO Committee on Pesticides in Agriculture
and the WHO Expert Committee on Pesticide Residues. FAO Meeting
Report, No.PL:1963/13: WHO/Food Add./23 (1964).

FAO/WHO.
1965a
Evaluation of the toxicity of pesticide residues in food. Report
of the Second Joint Meeting of the FAO Committee on Pesticides in
Agriculture and the WHO Expert Committee on Pesticide Residues.
FAO Meeting Report, No.PL:1965/10: WHO Food Add./26.65.

FAO/WHO.
1965b
Evaluation of the toxicity of pesticide residues in food. FAO
Meeting Report, No.PL:1965/10/1: WHO Food Add./27.65.

FAO/WHO.
1965c
Evaluation of the hazards to consumers resulting from the use of
fumigants in the protection of food. FAO Meeting Report,
No.PL:1965/10/2: WHO Food Add./28.65.

FAO/WHO.
1967a
Pesticide residues in food. Joint report of the FAO Working Party
on Pesticide Residues and the WHO Expert Committee on Pesticide
Residues. FAO Agricultural Studies, No. 73: WHO Technical Report
Series, No. 370.

FAO/WHO.
1967b
Evaluation of some pesticide residues in food. FAO:PL/CP/15: WHO
Food Add./67.32.

FAO/WHO.
1968a
Pesticide residues. Report of the 1967 Joint Meeting of the FAO
Working Party and the WHO Expert Committee. FAO Meeting Report,
No.PL:1967/M/11: WHO Technical Report Series, No. 391.

FAO/WHO.
1968b
1967 evaluation of some pesticide residues in food. FAO
PL:1967/M/11/1: WHO Food Add./68.30.

FAO/WHO.
1969a
Pesticide residues in food. Report of the 1968 Joint Meeting of
the FAO Working Party of Experts on Pesticide Residues and the WHO
Expert Committee on Pesticide Residues. FAO Agricultural Studies,
No. 78: WHO Technical Report Series, No. 417.

FAO/WHO.
1969b
1968 evaluation of some pesticide residues in food. FAO
PL:1968/M/9/1: WHO Food Add./69.35.

FAO/WHO.
1970a
Pesticide residues in food. Report of the 1969 Joint Meeting of the FAO Working Party of Experts on Pesticide Residues and the WHO Expert Group on Pesticide Residues. FAO Agricultural Studies, No. 84: WHO Technical Report Series, No. 458.

FAO/WHO.
1970b
1969 evaluations of some pesticide residues in food. FAO PL:1969/M/17: WHO Food Add./70.38.

FAO/WHO.
1971a
Pesticide residues in food. Report of the 1970 Joint Meeting of the FAO Working Party of Experts on Pesticide Residues. FAO Agricultural Studies, No. 87: WHO Technical Report Series, No. 474.

FAO/WHO.
1971b
1970 evaluations of some pesticide residues in food. AGP: 1970/M/12/1: WHO Food Add./71.42.

FAO/WHO.
1972a
Pesticide residues in food. Report of the 1971 Joint Meeting of the FAO Working Party of Experts on Pesticide Residues and the WHO Expert Committee on Pesticide Residues. FAO Agricultural Studies, No. 88: WHO Technical Report Series, No. 502.

FAO/WHO.
1972b
1971 evaluations of some pesticide residues in food. AGP: 1971/M/9/1: WHO Pesticide Residues Series, No. 1.

FAO/WHO.
1973a
Pesticide residues in food. Report of the 1972 Joint Meeting of the FAO Working Party of Experts on Pesticide Residues and the WHO Expert Committee on Pesticide Residues. FAO Agricultural Studies, No. 90: WHO Technical Report Series, No. 525.

FAO/WHO.
1973b
1972 evaluations of some pesticide residues in food. AGP: 1972/M/9/1: WHO Pesticide Residues Series, No. 2.

FAO/WHO.
1974a
Pesticide residues in food. Report of the 1973 Joint Meeting of the FAO Working Party of Experts on Pesticide Residues and the WHO Expert Committee on Pesticide Residues. FAO Agricultural Studies, No. 92: WHO Technical Report Series, No. 545.

FAO/WHO.
1974b
1973 evaluations of some pesticide residues in food. AGP: 1973/M/9/1: WHO Pesticide Residues Series, No. 3.

FAO/WHO.
1975a
Pesticide residues in food. Report of the 1974 Joint Meeting of the FAO Working Party of Experts on Pesticide Residues and the WHO Expert Committee on Pesticide Residues. FAO Agricultural Studies, No. 97: WHO Technical Report Series, No. 574.

FAO/WHO.
1975b
1974 evaluations of some pesticide residues in food. AGP: 1974/M/11: WHO Pesticide Residues Series, No. 4.

FAO/WHO.
1976
Pesticide residues in food. Report of the 1975 Joint Meeting of the FAO Working Party of Experts on Pesticide Residues. FAO Plant Production and Protection Series, No. 1: WHO Technical Report Series, No. 592.

FAO/WHO.
1977a
Pesticide residues in food. Report of the 1976 Joint Meeting of the FAO Panel of Experts on Pesticide Residues and the Environment and the WHO Expert Group on Pesticide Residues. FAO Food and Nutrition Series, No. 9. FAO Plant Production and Protection Series, No. 8: WHO Technical Report Series, No. 612.

FAO/WHO.
1977b
1976 evaluations of some pesticide residues in food. AGP: 1976/M/14.

FAO/WHO.
1978a
Pesticide residues in food. Report of the 1977 Joint Meeting of the FAO Panel of Experts on Pesticide Residues and the Environment and the WHO Expert Group on Pesticide Residues. FAO Plant Production and Protection Paper 10 Rev.

FAO/WHO.
1978b
1977 evaluations of some pesticide residues in food. FAO Plant Production and Protection Paper 10 Sup.

FAO/WHO.
1979a
Pesticide residues in food. Report of the 1978 Joint Meeting of the FAO Panel of Experts on Pesticide Residues in Food and the Environment and the WHO Expert Group on Pesticide Residues. FAO Plant Production and Protection Paper 15.

FAO/WHO.
1979b
1978 evaluations of some pesticide residues in food. FAO Plant Production and Protection Paper 15 Sup.

FAO/WHO.
1980a
Pesticide residues in food. Report of the 1979 Joint Meeting of the FAO Panel of Experts on Pesticide Residues in Food and the Environment and the WHO Expert Group on Pesticide Residues. FAO Plant Production and Protection Paper 20.

FAO/WHO.
1980b
1979 evaluations of some pesticide residues in food. FAO Plant Production and Protection Paper 20 Sup.

FAO/WHO.
1981a
Pesticide residues in food. Report of the 1980 Joint Meeting of the FAO Panel of Experts on Pesticide Residues in Food and the Environment and the WHO Expert Group on Pesticide Residues. FAO Plant Production and Protection Paper 26.

FAO/WHO.
1981b
1980 evaluations of some pesticide residues in food. FAO Plant Production and Protection Paper 26 Sup.

FAO/WHO.
1982
Pesticide residues in food. Report of the 1981 Joint Meeting of the FAO Panel of Experts on Pesticide Residues in Food and the Environment and the WHO Expert Group on Pesticide Residues. FAO Plant Production and Protection Paper 37.

FAO/WHO.
1982b
1981 evaluations of some pesticide residues in food. FAO Plant Production and Protection Paper 42.

FAO/WHO.
1983a
Pesticide residues in food. Report of the 1982 Joint Meeting of the FAO Panel of Experts on Pesticide Residues in Food and the Environment and the WHO Expert Group on Pesticide Residues. FAO Plant Production and Protection Paper 46.

FAO/WHO.   1982 evaluations of some pesticide residues in food. FAO Plant
1983b   Production and Protection Paper 49.

FAO/WHO.   Pesticide residues in food. Report of the 1983 Joint Meeting of
1984a   the FAO Panel of Experts on Pesticide Residues in Food and the
            Environment and the WHO Expert Group on Pesticide Residues. FAO
            Plant Production and Protection Paper 56.

FAO/WHO.   1983 evaluations of some pesticide residues in food. FAO Plant
1984b   Production and Protection Paper 61.

FAO/WHO.   Pesticide residues in food. Report of the 1984 Joint Meeting of
1985a   the FAO Panel of Experts on Pesticide Residues in Food and the
            Environment and the WHO Expert Group on Pesticide Residues. FAO
            Plant Production and Protection Paper 62.

FAO/WHO.   1984 evaluations of some pesticide residues in food. FAO Plant
1985b   Production and Protection Paper.

ANNEX I

ACCEPTABLE DAILY INTAKES, RESIDUE LIMITS AND GUIDELINE LEVELS
PROPOSED AT THE 1985 MEETING

These figures are additional to, or amend, those recorded in Annexes of the reports of earlier meetings. Limits recommended at meetings from 1965-1977 inclusive are summarized in document FAO/WHO 1978c.

This table includes maximum acceptable daily intake (ADIs), maximum residue limits (MRLs) and guideline levels (GLs). These terms are defined in Annex 3 of the report of the 1975 meeting. Part 1 lists ADIs and MRLs. Some ADIs and MRLs are temporary: in these cases the year in which further data are required is specified in parenthesis below the ADI and/or following the MRL(s). Part 2 lists GLs.

New, as distinct from amended, recommendations are identified by the symbol * before the commodity or before the ADI. Residue levels at or about the limit of determination are followed by the symbol **. Amended recommendations are followed by the previous recommendation in parenthesis.

The table includes the Codex Classification Numbers (CCNs) of both the compounds and the commodities listed, to facilitate reference to the Guide to Codex Maximum Limits for Pesticide Residues. CCNs for commodities are those of the revised Classificaton (see section 2.7).

PART I - ACCEPTABLE DAILY INTAKES (ADIs) AND MAXIMUM RESIDUE LIMITS (MRLs)

Pesticides, CCN and years of previous Evaluations	Recommended maximum ADI (mg/kg body weight)	Commodity		Recommended MRL or ERL (mg/kg)
		CCN	Name	
aldicarb CCN 117 1979, 1982	0.005	AS 0645	Maize forage	5 (fresh weight basis) (prev. 20 dry weight basis)

Remarks: MRLs are for the sum of aldicarb, its sulphoxide and its sulphone, expressed as aldicarb.

azocyclotin: See cyhexatin/azocyclotin.

captafol CCN 006 1969, 1973, 1974, 1976, 1977, 1982	Temporary ADI WITHDRAWN			All MRLs WITHDRAWN

Remarks: Temporary MRLs NOT replaced by GLs.

chlordimeform CCN 013 1971, 1975, 1977. 1978, 1979, 1980	0.0001 (1987)			

Remarks: Temporary ADI extended at the same level.

chlorothalonil CCN 081 1974, 1977, 1978, 1979, 1981, 1983	0.0005 (1987)	FB 0269	Grapes	10 (prev. 5)

Remarks: Temporary ADI extended at lower level. The limit for grapes remains temporary only because the ADI is temporary. TMRLs are for clorothalonil. Metabolites are not included.

cyhexatin CCN 067 1970, 1973, (as tri- cyclohexyltin hydroxide), 1974, 1975, 1977, 1978 , 1980, 1981, 1982, 1983	0.008	FP 0226	Apples	2[a,b]
		VP 0526	Beans	0.2[a,b]
		VO 0445	Bell peppers	0.5[a]
		FC 0001	Citrus fruits	2[a]
		VC 0424	Cucumbers	0.5[a]
		VO 0440	Egg plants	0.1**[b]
		VC 0425	Gherkins	1[a]
		FI 0328	Kiwi fruit	5[a]
		FB 0269	Grapes	2[b]
		MM 0095	Meat	0.2[a]
		VC 0046	Melons	0.5[a]
		ML 0812	Milk of cattle	0.05**[a]
			Milk products	0.05**[a]
		FS 0246	Peaches	5[a]
		FP 0230	Pears	2[a]
		FS 0014	Plums	2[a]
		FB 0275	Strawberries	2[a,b]
		DT 1114	Tea	2[a]
and		VO 0448	Tomatoes	2[a]
azocyclotin CN 129 1979, 1981, 1982, 1983	0.003			

[a] From good agricultural practice in the use of cyhexatin.
[b] From good agricultural practice in the use of azocyclotin.

Pesticides, CCN and years of previous Evaluations	Recommended maximum ADI (mg/kg body weight)	Commodity		Recommended MRL or ERL (mg/kg)
		CCN	Name	

Remarks: MRLs replace separate lists for the two compounds. They are numerically unchanged. MRLs are for the sum of azocyclotin (when azocyclotin has been applied), cyhexatin and dicyclohexyltin oxide expressed as cyhexatin.

cypermethrin CCN 118 1979, 1981, 1982, 1983, 1984	0.05	SO 0089 SO 0697 VD 0541	Oilseeds except peanuts Peanuts Soybeans	0.2 0.05** 0.05**

Remarks: MRLs are for cypermethrin (sum of isomers). Metabolites are not included. The MRL of 0.2 mg/kg previously applied to oilseeds, which did not include peanuts in the original Codex Classification. The MRLs for peanuts and soybeans replace the MRL for legume oilseeds at the same level.

deltamethrin CCN 135 1980, 1981, 1982, 1984	0.01	SB 0721	Coffee beans	0.02 (prev. 2)

Remarks: The change is to correct an error in the 1980 report and evaluations. MRLs are for deltamethrin. Metabolites are not included.

dichlofluanid CCN 082 1969, 1974, 1977, 1979, 1981, 1982 1983	0.3	DH 1100 CG 0640 CG 0647 CG 0650 CG 0654	Hops, dry Barley Oats Rye Wheat	MRL WITHDRAWN (prev. 1) 0.1)(prev. 0.1) 0.1 for 0.1) cereal 0.1) grains)

Remarks: MRLs are for dichlofluanid. Metabolites are not included.

diflubenzuron CCN 130 1981, 1983, 1984	0.02			

Remarks: Temporary ADI replaced by ADI at higher level. TMRLs replaced by MRLs. MRLs are for diflubenzuron. Metabolites are not included.

dimethipin CCN 151	*0.003 (1987)	SO 0691 SO 0495 SO 0702 VR 0589	*Cottonseed *Flaxseed *Rapeseed *Sunflower seed *Potatoes	0.5) 0.2) 0.1) (1987) 0.2) 0.1**)

Remarks: TMRLs are for dimethipin. Metabolites are not included. All limits are temporary pending receipt of the required information, irrespective of the status of the ADI.

dithiocarbamate fungicides CCN 105 1965, 1967, 1970, 1974, 1977, 1980, 1983(propineb and thiram), 1984(propineb and thiram)		VL 0482	*Lettuce, head-	5

Remarks: Limits are for residues determined and expressed as CS_2. Limits no longer apply to propineb or thiram because their temporary ADIs were withdrawn by this meeting. TMRLs for propineb are withdrawn; those for thiram are replaced by GLs.

Pesticides, CCN and years of previous Evaluations	Recommended maximum ADI (mg/kg body weight)	Commodity		Recommended MRL or ERL (mg/kg)
		CCN	Name	
endosulfan CCN 032 1965, 1967, 1968, 1971, 1974, 1975, 1982	0.008 (1989)			

Remarks: Temporary ADI extended at same level.

ethion CCN 034 1968, 1969, 1970, 1972, 1975, 1982, 1983	0.0005 (1986)			

Remarks: Temporary ADI extended at lower level.

fenamiphos CCN 085 1974, 1977, 1978, 1980	0.0003 (1987)			

Remarks: ADI replaced by temporary ADI at lower level. MRLs replaced by TMRLs.

fenvalerate CCN 119 1979, 1981, 1982, 1984	0.02 (1986)	SO 0697 VD 0541 ML 0812	Peanuts Soybeans Milk of cattle	0.1 0.1 0.1 (prev.0.01)

Remarks: TMRLs are for fenvalerate. Metabolites are not included. The recommendation for milk was omitted in 1984. The TMRLs for peanuts and soybeans replace the TMRL for legume oilseeds at the same level.

flucythrinate CCN 152	*0.02	FP 0009	*Pome fruits	0.5
		FB 0269	*Grapes	1
		FS 0246	*Peaches	0.5
		VS 0620	*Artichokes	0.5
		VD 0071	*Beans(dry)	0.5
		VB 0400) VB 0404)	*Brassicas,flower- head(broccoli, cauliflower)	0.2
		VB 0041	*Cabbages, head(Brussels sprouts; green, red, white, savoy cabbages)	0.2
		VD 0561	*Peas, field(dry)	0.05**
		VR 0589	*Potatoes	0.05**
		VR 0591	*Radish, Japanese	0.05**
		VR 0596	*Sugar beet	0.05**
		AV 0596	*Sugar beet leaves	2
		VO 0448	*Tomatoes	0.2
		CG 0640	*Barley	0.2
		CG 0647	*Oats	0.2
		CG 0654	*Wheat	0.2
		AS 0640	*Barley straw and fodder, dry	5
		AS 0647	*Oat straw and fodder, dry	5
		AS 0654	*Wheat straw and fodder, dry	5
		AF 0645	*Maize forage(green)	0.2

Pesticides, CCN and years of previous Evaluations	Recommended maximum ADI (mg/kg body weight)	Commodity		Recommended MRL or ERL (mg/kg)
		CCN	Name	
flucythrinate(cont'd)		SO 0691	*Cotton seed	0.1
		SO 0495	*Rapeseed	0.05**
		SB 0721	*Coffee beans	0.05**
		DT 1114	*Tea,dry manufactured	20
		DH 1100	*Hops, dry	10
		MM 0812	*Cattle meat	0.5(in the fat)
		MM 0814	*Goat meat	0.5(in the fat)
		ML 0812	*Milk of cattle	0.1
		PE 0112	*Eggs of poultry	0.05**

Remarks: Limits are for flucythrinate. Metabolites are not included. Limits
for cattle meat, goat meat, milk of cattle and eggs of poultry are
temporary until required information is provided.

Pesticides, CCN and years of previous Evaluations	Recommended maximum ADI	Commodity		Recommended MRL or ERL
imazalil CCN 110 1977, 1980, 1984	0.01 (1986)	FS 0012	*Stone fruits	5

Remarks: Temporary ADI extended at same level. TMRLs are for imazalil.
Metabolites are not included.

Pesticides, CCN and years of previous Evaluations	Recommended maximum ADI
mecarbam CCN 124	0.0005 (1986)

Remarks: Temporary ADI extended at lower level.

Pesticides, CCN and years of previous Evaluations	Recommended maximum ADI	Commodity		Recommended MRL or ERL
metalaxyl CCN 138 1982, 1984	0.03	FP 0226	*Apples	0.05**)
		FI 0311	Avocados	0.05**) (prev.0.1**))
		VB 0402	*Brussels sprouts	0.2)
		FB 0269	Grapes	2)(1986) (prev. 5))
		SO 0691	*Cottonseed	0.05**)
		FI 0341	*Pineapples(flesh)	0.05**)
		VD 0541	*Soybeans	0.1)
		FB 0275	*Strawberries	0.2)

Remarks: MRLs are for metalaxyl. Metabolites are not included. All MRLs are
temporary pending evaluation of data based on improved analytical
method.

Pesticides, CCN and years of previous Evaluations	Recommended maximum ADI
methamidophos CCN 100 1976, 1979, 1981, 1982, 1984	0.0006

Remarks: Temporary ADI replaced by ADI at slightly higher level. TMRLs
replaced by MRLs.

Pesticides, CCN and years of previous Evaluations	Recommended maximum ADI
methiocarb CCN 132 1981, 1983	0.001

Remarks: The withdrawal by the 1983 meeting of the MRLs for apples, blueberries,
cherries, currants (red), grapes and peaches is now confirmed.

Pesticides, CCN and years of previous Evaluations	Recommended maximum ADI (mg/kg body weight)	Commodity		Recommended MRL or ERL (mg/kg)
		CCN	Name	

omethoate
CCN 055
1971, 1975, 1978,
1979, 1981, 1984

	0.0003			

<u>Remarks</u>: Temporary ADI replaced by ADI at slightly lower level. TMRLs replaced
by MRLs.

oxamyl
CCN 126
1980, 1983, 1984

	0.03	FC 0001	Citrus fruits	5 (prev. 3)
		VP 0526	Beans, kidney	5 (prev. 3)
		VP 0534	Beans, Lima	5 (prev. 3)
		VD 0526	Beans, kidney(dry)	0.05**(1986)
		VS 0624	Celery	5 (prev. 3)
		VC 0424	Cucumbers	2 (prev.0.5)
		VO 0445	Pepper, bell	2 (prev.3 for peppers)
		VR 0075	*Root and tuber vegetables	0.1

<u>Remarks</u>: MRLs are for the sum of oxamyl and its oxime, expressed as oxamyl.
The level of the limit for kidney beans(dry) is confirmed, but the
limit remains temporary pending confirmation of nationally approved
uses. Limit for root and tuber vegetables replaces individual limits
at same level for sugar beets, beets, carrots, potatoes and sweet
potatoes.

paraquat
CCN 057
1970, 1972, 1976,
1978, 1981, 1982

	0.001 (1986)			

<u>Remarks</u>: Temporary ADI extended at same level. It refers to paraquat dichloride

2-phenylphenol
CCN 056
1969, 1975, 1983

	0.02 (1989)			

<u>Remarks</u>: Temporary ADI extended at same level.

phorate
CCN 112
1977, 1982, 1983,
1984

	0.0002			

<u>Remarks</u>: Temporary ADI replaced by ADI at same level. TMRLs replaced by MRLs.

phosphamidon
CCN 061
1965, 1966, 1968,
1969, 1972, 1974,
1982

	0.0005 (1986)			

<u>Remarks</u>: Temporary ADI extended at lower level.

Pesticides, CCN and years of previous Evaluations	Recommended maximum ADI (mg/kg body weight)	Commodity		Recommended MRL or ERL (mg/kg)
		CCN	Name	
pirimiphos-methyl CCN 086 1974, 1976, 1977, 1979, 1983	0.01	FC 0001	Citrus fruits	2 (prev.0.5)
		MD 0180	*Dried fish	10
		SO 0697	Peanuts(whole)	25 (prev.50)
		SO 0697	Peanuts(kernels)	2 (prev. 5)
		OR	Peanut oil	15 (prev.10)

Remarks: MRLs are for pirimiphos-methyl. Metabolites are not included.

Pesticides, CCN and years of previous Evaluations	Recommended maximum ADI	Commodity		Recommended MRL or ERL
		CCN	Name	
prochloraz CCN 142 1983	0.01	CG 0640	Barley	0.5 (prev.0.05**[a])
		CG 0647	Oats	0.5 (prev.0.05**[a])
		CG 0650	Rye	0.5 (prev.0.05**[a])
		CG 0654	Wheat	0.5 (prev.0.05**[a])
		AS 0640	Barley straw and fodder, dry	15 (prev.0.2[a])
		AS 0647	Oat straw and fodder, dry	15 (prev.0.2[a])
		AS 0650	Rye straw and fodder, dry	15 (prev.0.2[a])
		AS 0654	Wheat straw and fodder, dry	15 (prev.0.2[a])
			Mushrooms	2
		FC 0001	Citrus fruits	5(TMRL) (prev. 5[a])
		MM 0812	*Cattle meat	0.1**(TMRL)
		MM 0812	*Cattle meat	0.1**(TMRL) (in the fat)
		MO 0812	*Edible offal of cattle	2(TMRL)
		ML 0812	*Milk of cattle	0.1**(TMRL)

[a] Previous limits were for prochlorate only.

Remarks: MRLs for all commodities are now for the sum of prochloraz and its
metabolites containing the 2,4,6-trichlorophenol moiety, expressed
as prochloraz. TMRLs for citrus fruits and animal products are
temporary until required information is provided. Previously
proposed TMRLs for avocado, banana, mango and rapeseed are no longer
temporary. Those for stone fruits and papaya remain temporary. MRLs
for avocado and mango cover cumulative residues from pre- and post-
harvest treatments.

Pesticides, CCN and years of previous Evaluations	Recommended maximum ADI	Commodity		Recommended MRL or ERL
propineb CN 105 (dithiocarbamates) 1977, 1980, 1983, 1984	Temporary ADI WITHDRAWN			All TMRLs WITHDRAWN

Remarks: TMRLs for propineb are NOT replaced by GLs. GLs for propylenethiourea
(PTU) are withdrawn.

Pesticides, CCN and years of previous Evaluations	Recommended maximum ADI (mg/kg body weight)	Commodity		Recommended MRL or ERL (mg/kg)
		CCN	Name	
pyrazophos CCN 153	no ADI See Part 2.			
thiodicarb CCN 154	*0.01 (1987)	SO 0691	*Cottonseed	0.5
		OR 0691	*Cottonseed oil (refined)	0.02**
		VD 0541	*Soybeans	0.2
		OR 0541	*Soybean oil(refined)	0.02**
		CG 0654	*Maize	0.05**
		AS 0645	*Maize fodder	50
		AF 0645	*Maize forage	50
		VO 0447	*Sweet corn	2
		VO 0448	*Tomatoes	1
		MM 0812	*Cattle meat	0.02**
		ML 0812	*Milk of cattle	0.02**

Remarks: TMRLs are for the sum of thiodicarb, methomyl and methyl hydroxy-thioacetimidate("methomyloxime"), expressed as thiodicarb.

thiram CCN 105 (dithiocarbamates) 1965, 1967, 1970, 1974, 1977, 1983, 1984	Temporary ADI WITHDRAWN			

Remarks: TMRLs converted to GLs. See Part 2.

triadimefon CCN 133 1979, 1981, 1983, 1984	0.03			

Remarks: Temporary ADI replaced by ADI at higher level. TMRLs replaced by MRLs.

vamidothion CCN 078 1973, 1982	0.0003 (1988)	VB 0402	Brussels sprouts	Withdrawn (prev. 1)
		FP 0009	*Pome fruits	1
		FS 0246	*Peaches	0.5
		CG 0080	*Cereal grains,including rice(hulled)	0.2

Remarks: Temporary ADI extended at same level. TMRLs are for the sum of vamidothion, its sulphoxide and its sulphone, expressed as vamidothion. The limit for pome fruits replaces separate limits of 2 mg/kg for apples and pears.

PART 2 - GUIDELINE LEVELS (NO ACCEPTABLE DAILY INTAKES)

Pesticide,CCN and years of previous Evaluations	Commodity		Guideline level (mg/kg)
	CCN	Name	
binapacryl	FC 0004	*Oranges	0.1
CCN 003	DH 1100	*Hops	0.5
1969, 1974, 1982			

Remarks: GLs are for binapacryl. Metabolites are not included.

dialifos
CCN 098
1976, 1982

Remarks: The definition of the residue in commodities of plant origin is
changed and is now identical to that in commodities of animal
origin: dialifos.

pyrazophos	FP 0226	*Apples	0.5
CCN 153	FB 0275	*Strawberries	0.2
	VB 0402	*Brussels sprouts	0.1
	VC 0424	*Cucumbers	0.1
	VC 0046	*Melons	0.1
	VR 0577	*Carrots	0.2
	CG 0640	*Barley	0.05
	CG 0654	*Wheat	0.05
	DH 1100	*Hops, dry	10

Remarks: GLs are for pyrazophos. Metabolites are not included.

thiram
CCN 105
(dithiocarbamates)
1965, 1967, 1970, 1974,
1977, 1983, 1984

Remarks: As the temporary ADI has been withdrawn, previously recommended
TMRLs are converted to GLs. The GLs are determined and expressed
as CS_2.

ANNEX IIA
**NEW MAXIMUM RESIDUE LIMITS RECOMMENDED AT THE 1985 MEETING
CLASSIFIED IN COMMODITY GROUPS**

CLASS A - PRIMARY FOOD COMMODITIES OF PLANT ORIGIN

01.　　<u>FRUITS</u>

002 POME FRUITS
FP	0009	Pome fruits	flucythrinate (0.5) vamidothion (1)
	0226	Apples	metalaxyl (0.05**)

003 STONE FRUITS
FS	0012	Stone fruits	imazalil (5)
	0246	Peaches	flucythrinate (0.5) vamidothion (0.5)

004 BERRIES AND OTHER SMALL FRUITS
FB	0269	Grapes	flucythrinate (1) metalaxyl (2)
FB	0275	Strawberries	metalaxyl (0.2)

006 ASSORTED TROPICAL AND SUB-TROPICAL FRUITS - INEDIBLE
　　 PEEL
FI	0311	Avocados	metalaxyl (0.05**)
FI	0341	Pineapples (flesh)	metalaxyl (0.05**)

02.　　<u>VEGETABLES</u>

010 BRASSICA (COLE OR CABBAGE) VEGETABLES
VB	0400)	Brassicas, flowerhead -	
VB	0404)	(broccoli, cauliflower)	flucythrinate (0.2)
VB	0041	Cabbages, head - (Brussels sprouts, green, red, white, savoy cabbage)	flucythrinate (0.2)
VB	0402	Brussels sprouts	metalaxyl (0.2)

012 FRUITING VEGETABLES, OTHER THAN CUCURBITS
VO	0448	Tomatoes	flucythrinate (0.2) thiodicarb (1)
VO	0447	Sweet corn	thiodicarb (2)

013 LEAFY VEGETABLES
VL   0482   Lettuce, head   dithiocarbamates (5)

015 PULSES
VD   0071   Beans (dry)   flucythrinate (0.5)
VD   0541   Soybeans   metalaxyl (0.1)
                                        thiodicarb (0.2)
VD   0561   Peas, field (dry)   flucythrinate (0.05**)

016 ROOT AND TUBER VEGETABLES
VR   0075   Root and tuber
             vegetables   oxamyyl (0.1)
VR   0539   Potatoes   dimethipin (0.1**)
                                        flucythrinate (0.05**)
VR   0589   Radish, Japanese   flucythrinate (0.05**)
VR   0596   Sugar beet   flucythrinate (0.05**)

017 STALK AND STEM VEGETABLES
VS   0620   Artichokes   flucythrinate (0.5)

03.   GRASSES

020 CEREAL GRAINS
CG   0080   Cereal grains (including
             rice, hulled)   vamidothion (0.2)
CG   0640   Barley   flucythrinate (0.2)
CG   0645   Maize   thiodicarb (0.05**)
CG   0647   Oats   flucythrinate (0.2)
CG   0654   Wheat   flucythrinate (0.2)

04.   NUTS AND SEEDS

023 OIL SEEDS
SO   0691   Cottonseed   dimethipin (0.5)
                                        flucythrinate (0.1)
                                        metataxyl (0.05**)
                                        thiodicarb (0.5)
-            Flaxseed   dimethipin (0.2)
SO   0495   Rapeseed   dimethipin (0.1)
                                        flucythrinate (0.05**)
SO   0702   Sunflower seed   dimethipin (0.2)

024 SEED FOR BEVERAGES AND SWEETS
SB   0721   Coffee beans   flucythrinate (0.05**)

CLASS B - PRIMARY FOOD COMMODITIES OF ANIMAL ORIGIN

06.   <u>MAMMALIAN PRODUCTS</u>

    030 MEATS (MAMMALIAN)

MM	0812	Cattle meat	flucythrinate (0.5 [in the fat])
			prochloraz (0.1**)
			prochloraz (0.1** [in the fat])
			thiodicarb (0.02**)
MM	0814	Goat meat	flucythrinate (0.5 [in the fat])

    032 EDIBLE OFFAL (MAMMALIAN)

| MO | 0812 | Edible offal of cattle | prochloraz (2) |

    033 MILKS

ML	0812	Cattle milk	flucythrinate (0.1)
			prochloraz (0.1**)
			thiodicarb (0.02**)

07.   <u>POULTRY PRODUCTS</u>

    039 EGGS

| PE | 0112 | Eggs (poultry) | flucythrinate (0.05**) |

CLASS C - PRIMARY ANIMAL FEED COMMODITIES

11.   <u>PRIMARY FOOD COMMODITIES OF PLANT ORIGIN</u>

    051 STRAW, FODDER AND FORAGE OF CEREAL GRAINS AND GRASSES (INCLUDING BUCKWHEAT FODDER)

AS	0640	Barley straw and fodder (dry)	flucythrinate (5)
AS	0647	Oat straw and fodder, dry	flucythrinate (5)
AS	0654	Wheat straw and fodder, dry	flucythrinate (5)
AF	0645	Maize fodder	thiodicarb (50)
AS	0645	Maize fodder (green)	flucythrinate (0.2)
			thiodicarb (50)

052 MISCELLANEOUS FODDER AND FORAGE CROPS
AV   0596   Sugarbeet leaves   flucythrinate (2)

CLASS D - PROCESSED FOODS OF PLANT ORIGIN

12.   SECONDARY FOOD COMMODITIES OF PLANT ORIGIN

057 DRIED HERBS
DH   1100   Hops, dry   flucythrinate (10)

13.   DERIVED PRODUCTS OF PLANT ORIGIN

066 TEAS
DT   1114   Tea (dry manufactured)   flucythrinate (20)

068 VEGETABLE OILS, EDIBLE (OR REFINED)
OR   0691   Cottonseed oil
             (refined)   thiodicarb (0.02**)
OR   0541   Soybean oil
             (refined)   thiodicarb (0.02**)

CLASS E - PROCESSED FOODS OF ANIMAL ORIGIN

16.   SECONDARY FOOD COMMODITIES OF ANIMAL ORIGIN

080 DRIED MEAT AND FISH PRODUCTS
MD   0180   Dried fish   pirimiphos-methyl (10)

ANNEX IIB

CHANGES IN MAXIMUM RESIDUE LIMITS
RECOMMENDED AT THE 1985 MEETING

		FROM	TO
Aldicarb	Maize forage	20 (dry weight basis)	5 (fresh weight basis)
Chlorothalonil	Grapes	5	10
Cypermethrin	Oilseeds	0.2	0.2 for oilseeds except peanuts
	Legume oilseeds	0.05**	0.05** for peanuts and soybeans
Deltamethrin	Coffee beans	2	0.02
Dichlofluanid	Cereal grains	0.1	0.1 for barley, oats, rye and wheat
	Hops, dry	1	withdrawn
Fenvalerate	Legume oilseeds	0.1	0.1 for peanuts and soybeans
	Milk	0.01	0.1
Metalaxyl	Avocados	0.1**	0.05**
	Grapes	5	2
Oxamyl	Citrus fruits	3	5
	Beans, kidney	3	5
	Beans, lima	3	5
	Celery	3	5
	Cucumbers	0.5	2
	Peppers	3	2 for peppers, bell
Pirimiphos-methyl	Citrus fruits	0.5	2
	Peanuts (whole)	50	25
	Peanuts (kernels)	5	2
	Peanut oil	10	15
Prochloraz	Barley	0.05**	0.5
	Oats	0.05**	0.5
	Rye	0.05**	0.5

Prochloraz
(Cont'd)

	FROM	TO
Wheat	0.05**	0.5
Barley straw	0.2	15
Oat straw	0.2	15
Rye straw	0.2	15
Wheat straw	0.2	15
Mushrooms	2	2
Citrus fruits	5	5

<u>Note</u>: previous MRLs were for prochloraz only. New MRLs are for sum of prochloraz and its metabolites containing the 2,4,5-trichlorophenol moiety, expressed as prochloraz.

ANNEX III

<u>FAO/WHO JOINT MEETING ON PESTICIDE RESIDUES</u>
<u>INDEX OF REPORTS AND EVALUATIONS</u>

ACEPHATE	1976, 1979, 1981, 1982, 1984	sec-BUTYLAMINE	1975, 1977, 1978, 1979, 1980, 1981, 1984 (withdrawal of TADI – no evaluation)
ALDICARB	1979, 1982, 1985		
ALDRIN	1976, 1966, 1967, 1974, 1975, 1977	CAMPHECHLOR	1968, 1973
ALLETHRIN	1965	CAPTAFOL	1969, 1973, 1974, 1976, 1977, 1982, 1985
AMINOCARB	1978, 1979		
AMITRAZ	1980, 1983, 1984, 1985	CAPTAN	1965, 1969, 1973, 1974, 1977, 1978, 1980, 1982, 1984
AMITROLE	1974, 1977		
AZINPHOSETHYL	1973, 1983	CARBARYL	1965, 1966, 1967, 1968, 1969, 1970, 1973, 1975, 1976, 1977, 1979, 1984
AZINPHOS-METHYL	1965, 1968, 1972, 1973, 1974		
AZOCYCLOTIN	1979, 1981, 1982, 1983, 1985	CARBENDAZIM	1973, 1976, 1977, 1978, 1983, 1985
BENDIOCARB	1982, 1984	CARBOFURAN	1976, 1979, 1980, 1982
BENOMYL	1973, 1975, 1983	CARBON DISULPHIDE	1965, 1967, 1968, 1971, 1985
BHC (technical) (see also lindane)	1965, 1968, 1973	CARBON TETRACHLORIDE	1965, 1967, 1968, 1971, 1979, 1985
BINAPACRYL	1969, 1974, 1982, 1984, 1985	CARBOPHENOTHION	1972, 1976, 1977, 1979, 1980, 1983
BIORESMETHRIN	1975, 1976	CARBOSULFAN	1984
BITERTANOL	1983, 1984	CARTAP	1976, 1978
BROMIDE ION	1968, 1969, 1971, 1979, 1981, 1983	CHINOMETHIONAT	1968, 1974, 1977, 1981, 1983, 1984
BROMOMETHANE	1966, 1967, 1968, 1971, 1979, 1985	CHLORBENSIDE	1965
BROMOPHOS	1972, 1975, 1977, 1982, 1984, 1985	CHLORDANE	1965, 1967, 1969, 1970, 1972, 1974, 1977, 1982, 1984
BROMOPHOS-ETHYL	1972, 1975, 1977	CHLORDIMEFORM	1971, 1975, 1977, 1978, 1979, 1980, 1985
BROMOPROPYLATE	1973	CHLORFENSON	1965
BUTOCARBOXIM	1983, 1985	CHLORFENVINPHOS	1971, 1984

CHLORMEQUAT	1970, 1972, 1976, 1985	DEMETON-S-METHYL and related compounds	1965, 1967, 1968, 1973, 1979, 1982, 1983, 1984
CHLOROBENZILATE	1965, 1968, 1972, 1975, 1977, 1980	DIALIFOS	1976, 1982, 1985
CHLOROPROPYLATE	1968, 1972	DIAZINON	1965, 1966, 1967, 1968, 1970, 1975, 1979
CHLOROTHALONIL	1974, 1977, 1978, 1979, 1981, 1983, 1984 (corrections to 1983 report), 1985	1,2 DIBROMO-ETHANE	1966, 1967, 1968, 1971, 1979, 1985
		DICHLOFLUANID	1969, 1974, 1977, 1979, 1981, 1982, 1983, 1985
CHLORPROPHAM	1965	1,2-DICHLORO-ETHANE	1967, 1971, 1979, 1985
CHLORPYRIFOS	1972, 1974, 1975, 1977, 1981, 1982, 1983	DICHLORVOS	1965, 1966, 1967, 1969, 1970, 1974, 1977
CHLORPYRIFOS-METHYL	1975, 1979	DICLORAN	1974, 1977
CHLORTHION	1965	DICOFOL	1968, 1970, 1974
COUMAPHOS	1968, 1972, 1975, 1978, 1983	DIELDRIN	1965, 1966, 1967, 1968, 1969, 1970, 1974, 1977
CRUFOMATE	1968, 1972	DIFLUBENZURON	1981, 1983, 1984, 1985
CYANOFENPHOS	1975, 1978 (ADI extended, but no evaluation), 1980, 1982, 1983	DIMETHIPIN	1985
		DIMETHOATE	1965, 1966, 1967, 1970, 1977, 1983, 1984
CYHALOTHRIN	1984		
CYHEXATIN (TRICYCLO= HEXYLTIN HYDROXIDE '70 & '73)	1970, 1973, 1974, 1975, 1977, 1978, 1980, 1981, 1982, 1983, 1985	DIMETHRIN	1965
		DINOCAP	1969, 1974
		DIOXATHION	1968, 1972
CYPERMETHRIN	1979, 1981, 1982, 1983, 1984, 1985	DIPHENYL	1966, 1967
		DIPHENYLAMINE	1969, 1976, 1979, 1982, 1984
2,4-D	1970, 1971, 1974, 1975, 1980, 1985		
DAMINOZIDE	1977, 1983	DIQUAT	1970, 1972, 1976, 1977, 1978
DDT	1965, 1966, 1967, 1968, 1969, 1979, 1980, 1983, 1984	DISULFOTON	1973, 1975, 1979, 1981, 1984
DELTAMETHRIN	1980, 1981, 1982, 1984, 1985	DITHIOCARBAMATE FUNGICIDES	1965, 1967, 1970, 1974, 1977, 1980, 1983, 1985
DEMETON	1965, 1967, 1975, 1982, 1983	DNOC	1965

DODINE	1974, 1976, 1977
EDIFENPHOS	1976, 1979, 1981
ENDOSULFAN	1965, 1967, 1968, 1971, 1974, 1975, 1982, 1985
ENDRIN	1965, 1970, 1974, 1975
ETHEPHON	1977, 1978, 1983, 1985
ETHIOFENCARB	1977, 1978, 1981, 1982, 1983
ETHION	1968, 1969, 1970, 1972, 1975, 1982, 1983
ETHOPROPHOS	1983, 1984
ETHOXYQUIN	1969
ETHYLENE OXIDE	1965, 1968, 1971
ETRIMFOS	1980, 1982
FENAMIPHOS	1974, 1977, 1978, 1980, 1985
FENBUTATIN OXIDE	1977, 1979
FENCHLORPHOS	1968, 1972, 1980 1983
FENITROTHION	1969, 1974, 1976, 1977, 1979, 1982, 1983, 1984
FENSULFOTHION	1972, 1982, 1983
FENTHION	1971, 1975, 1977, 1978, 1979, 1980, 1983
FENTIN compounds	1965, 1970, 1972
FENVALERATE	1979, 1981, 1982, 1984, 1985
FERBAM	see dithiocarbamate fungicides
FLUCYTHRINATE	1985
FOLPET	1969, 1973, 1974, 1982, 1984
FORMOTHION	1969, 1972, 1973
GUAZATINE	1978, 1980
HEPTACHLOR	1965, 1966, 1967, 1968, 1969, 1970, 1974, 1975, 1977
HEXACHLORO- BENZENE	1969, 1973, 1974, 1978, 1985
HYDROGEN CYANIDE	1965
HYDROGEN PHOSPHIDE	1965, 1966, 1967, 1969, 1971
IMAZALIL	1977, 1980, 1984, 1985
IPRODIONE	1977, 1980
ISOFENPHOS	1981, 1982, 1984, 1985
LEAD ARSENATE	1965, 1968
LEPTOPHOS	1974, 1975, 1978
LINDANE	1965, 1966, 1967, 1968, 1969, 1970, 1973, 1974, 1975, 1977, 1978, 1979
MALATHION	1965, 1966, 1967, 1968, 1969, 1970, 1973, 1975, 1977, 1984
MALEIC HYDRAZIDE	1976, 1977, 1980, 1984
MANEB	see dithiocarbamate fungicides
MANCOZEB	1967, 1970, 1974, 1977, 1980
MECARBAM	1980, 1983, 1985
METALAXYL	1982, 1984, 1985
METHACRIFOS	1980, 1982
METHAMIDOPHOS	1976, 1979, 1981, 1982, 1984, 1985
METHIDATHION	1972, 1975, 1979
METHIOCARB	1981, 1983, 1984, 1985
METHOMYL	1975, 1976, 1977, 1978
METHOPRENE	1984

METHOXYCHLOR	1965, 1977
METHYL BROMIDE	see bromomethane
MEVINPHOS	1965, 1972
MGK 264	1967
MONOCROTOPHOS	1972, 1975
NABAM	see dithiocarbamate fungicides
NITROFEN	1983
OMETHOATE	1971, 1975, 1978, 1979, 1981, 1984, 1985
ORGANOMERCURY	1965, 1966, 1967
OXAMYL	1980, 1983, 1984, 1985
OXYDEMETON-METHYL	1965, 1967, 1968, 1973, 1984
OXYTHIOQUINOX	see chinomethionat
PARAQUAT	1970, 1972, 1976, 1978, 1981, 1982, 1985
PARATHION	1965, 1967, 1969, 1970, 1984
PARATHION-METHYL	1965, 1968, 1972, 1975, 1978, 1979, 1980, 1982, 1984
PERMETHRIN	1979, 1980, 1981, 1982, 1983, 1984
2-PHENYLPHENOL	1969, 1975, 1983, 1985
PHENOTHRIN	1979, 1980, 1982, 1984
PHENTHOATE	1980, 1981, 1984
PHORATE	1977, 1982, 1983, 1984, 1985
PHOSALONE	1972, 1975, 1976
PHOSMET	1976, 1977, 1978, 1979, 1981, 1984, 1985
PHOSPHAMIDON	1965, 1966, 1968, 1969, 1972, 1974, 1982
PHOXIM	1982, 1983, 1984
PIPERONYL BUTOXIDE	1965, 1966, 1967, 1969, 1972
PIRIMICARB	1976, 1978, 1979, 1981, 1982, 1985
PIRIMIPHOS-METHYL	1974, 1976, 1977, 1979, 1983, 1985
PROCHLORAZ	1983, 1985
PROCYMIDONE	1981, 1982
PROPAMOCARB	1984
PROPARGITE	1977, 1978, 1979, 1980, 1982
PROPHAM	1965
PROPINEB	1977, 1980, 1983, 1984, 1985
PROPOXUR	1973, 1981, 1983
PYRAZOPHOS	1985
PYRETHRINS	1965, 1966, 1967, 1968, 1969, 1970, 1972, 1974
QUINTOZENE	1969, 1973, 1974, 1975, 1977
2,4,5-T	1970, 1979, 1981
TECNAZENE	1974, 1978, 1981, 1983
THIABENDAZOLE	1970, 1971, 1972, 1975, 1977, 1979, 1981
THIODICARB	1985
THIOMETON	1969, 1973, 1976, 1979
THIOPHANATE-METHYL	1973, 1975, 1977
THIRAM	see dithiocarbamate fungicides 1983, 1984, 1985
TOXAPHENE	see camphechlor
TRIADIMEFON	1979, 1981, 1983, 1984, 1985

TRIAZOPHOS	1982, 1983, 1984 (corrections to 1983 report)	TRIFORINE	1977, 1978
		VAMIDOTHION	1973, 1982, 1985
TRICHLORFON	1971, 1975, 1978	ZINEB	see dithiocarbamate fungicides
TRICHLORONAT	1971		
TRICHLORO-ETHYLENE	1968	ZIRAM	see dithiocarbamate fungicides